Denise's

DAILY
DOZEN

The Easy, Every Day Program

to Lose Up to

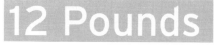 12 Pounds

in 2 Weeks

DENISE AUSTIN

CENTER
STREET®

NEW YORK BOSTON NASHVILLE

Exercise photos by Hilmar Meyer-Bosse

Center Street
Hachette Book Group
237 Park Avenue
New York, NY 10017

www.centerstreet.com

Center Street is a division of Hachette Book Group, Inc.
The Center Street name and logo are trademarks of Hachette Book Group, Inc.

Printed in the United States of America

First Edition: January 2010
10 9 8 7 6 5 4 3 2 1

Library of Congress Cataloging-in-Publication Data
Austin, Denise.
    Denise's daily dozen : the easy, every day program to lose up to 12 pounds in 2 weeks /
Denise Austin—1st ed.
       p.   cm.
Includes index.
ISBN 978-1-59995-244-4
1. Reducing diets.   2. Weight loss.
   RM222.2 .A878 2010
   613.2/5—dc22   2009021019

With the most humble of hearts for the blessing of such a wonderful family and upbringing, I dedicate this book to my mom and dad, whom I miss every day.

CONTENTS

ACKNOWLEDGMENTS

want to thank *all* my loving family . . . each one, from the oldest to the youngest. We are truly blessed to have such a close-knit big family. I treasure all of our times together.

I'm so thankful to my husband, Jeff, for our happy life together . . . twenty-five years of your amazing love, loyalty, and laughter. I have tears in my eyes of pure pride and gratefulness for our daughters, Kelly and Katie, who have both grown up to be such hardworking, caring, and "love of life" people. I'm so proud to be your mom.

I want to thank Michele Bender for all her help with this book. You are a joy to work with. Also, thanks to Christopher Mohr, PhD, RD, CSSD, a sports nutritionist, for all his help planning healthy meals. A big thanks to all my friends at Hachette, especially Harry Helm and my book editor, Christina Boys.

A very special thank-you to Jan Miller and Nena Madonia, for everything!

Thanks to my three sisters and my great bunch of girlfriends who are so supportive and always there for me, helping me with some of the recipes and testing some of these exercises.

I love what I do, helping people to feel better about themselves and making a positive difference in their lives.

—Denise Austin

INTRODUCTION

People always ask me where I get all my energy. It's true that at fifty-two years old I have more energy than I did at twenty-two! I feel great, too (and I'm proud to say I'm 100 percent all natural). It's a direct result of a well-rounded lifestyle that includes everything from fitness to healthy eating to stress reduction to sleep and more. I want you to feel good, too, and get through your day with energy. I want you to change your lifestyle so that you wake up and start each day on a healthier and happier foot. You can have all the money in the world, but if you don't have your health, you have nothing.

In this book, I'll share all my secrets and tips for living your healthiest lifestyle ever. But it goes beyond my own experience and expertise I am a curious person, and I spend a lot of time asking the most brilliant people in the world a lot of questions. It's true. Thanks to the work that I do with the President's Council on Physical Fitness and Sports, I am surrounded by some of the top experts in our country from world-renowned organizations like the Mayo Clinic, Cooper Clinic, National Institutes of Health, and more. I talk to these experts on a regular basis, querying them on the latest news, research, and what's in store for the future. In other words, I have done a lot of information gathering for you and am excited to pass it on because I want to help you live a fitter, healthier, and more enjoyable life. I know that what you want is simple, reliable information that is quick and easy. I know this from my thirty years in the health and fitness industry, but I also know it because that's exactly what *I* want. I'm a wife and a mother and understand what it's like to work full-time and juggle all the responsibilities

Be fit, healthy, and happy forever . . .

of a family. But despite a busy life, you *can* look and feel your best. In *Denise's Daily Dozen*, I've compiled the newest health information so that you can reap all the benefits. Remember, you only live once; why not live it as healthy and vibrantly as you can?

PART ONE

GETTING READY

The Daily Dozen Fitness Plan

Do you want to boost your metabolism, burn fat, tone up, and get in the best shape of your life? Good! That's just what the Daily Dozen Fitness Plan is going to do! Each day, you'll have twelve easy exercises that you can do in twelve minutes. In just two weeks, you can lose up to twelve pounds! I've designed these exercises to blast fat, burn calories, shrink your fat zones, and help you tone up. Each day's routine makes the most out of those twelve minutes so you are training smarter in a short amount of time. But I'm not just *saying* this works; I *know* it does. Why? Because this is how I keep my own weight down and stay firm. Fitness may be my day job, but that doesn't mean I want to spend all day working out. I don't. Instead, I maximize every minute of my workouts doing compound exercises that target more than one muscle group at a time and combining cardio workouts with toning. And that's exactly the program that I've designed for you with the Daily Dozen Fitness Plan.

Your Daily Dozen: Twelve Easy Exercises in Twelve Minutes a Day

To me, there are three main components of a well-balanced workout: cardiovascular exercise, toning, and flexibility. Each one is important, and the Daily Dozen includes them all.

Cardiovascular exercise is critical for burning calories and melting fat off your body as well as keeping your heart muscle healthy. Cardio exercise blasts off fat, shedding pounds. It also boosts your fitness level so you can do things like climb stairs without huffing and puffing. My favorite form of cardio exercise is walking—and it's also one of the easiest! It's great for your legs and relieving stress, but the reason I really love walking is that you can do it almost anywhere, and anyone can do it.

Toning exercises firm all the muscles in your body, including your abs, arms, buttocks, thighs, hips, chest, shoulders, and back. Toning through strength training, using both free weights and your own body weight, is also important for slimming down, because the more muscles you build, the more you boost your metabolism. The reason? Muscle demands more energy from your body than fat does. So the more muscle you add to your body, the more calories you'll be burning throughout the day. In fact, studies show that for every pound of muscle you add, you automatically burn an extra thirty-five to fifty calories per day—and that's while going about your normal activities. Even at rest, muscle burns almost twice as many calories as fat. (Isn't that amazing?)

Now, I know some women are hesitant about strength training with weights because they're afraid they'll look too bulked up or masculine. But it's time to

Actions speak louder than words. Walk and talk!

change that thinking! Men typically develop big, bulky muscles because of the high level of the hormone testosterone that they have in their bodies. Though women's bodies have some testosterone, too, it's not nearly enough to get those bulging muscles. So don't worry about the exercises in the Daily Dozen bulking you up. They won't. Rather, these strength moves tighten and tone and eventually redistribute your weight in a healthy way. Your arms and legs will feel firmer, your body will feel stronger, and you'll be burning more calories daily—even when you're sleeping!

The third essential element of a well-balanced fitness program is flexibility. As we age, we naturally lose flexibility, so we've got to do a little work in order to stay agile and spry and continue walking with a spring in our steps. Flexibility wards off injuries from exercising as well as day-to-day activities. For example, how many times have you heard about people throwing their backs out simply by reaching for something or picking something up? Maybe you've experienced this yourself. But increasing flexibility can prevent injuries just like this. Of course, stretching is also very relaxing, helping you release tension—especially in your hips and back—and simply makes you feel better. That's why we warm up before and stretch at the end of every workout in the Daily Dozen, and it's why I've included a yoga routine.

The Daily Dozen Fitness Plan contains all three elements—cardiovascular, toning, and flexibility—in the twelve easy moves you do for twelve minutes each day. By the end of the week, you've done them all!

In addition to sculpting your muscles, blasting flab, and boosting flexibility, all of these workouts will help shrink your fat cells. We're each born with a set number of fat cells, so it's not the number that makes us, well, fat; it's how big they get. Several things impact the size of your fat cells, and two of the big ones are exercise and eating. By exercising and eating right, you're helping to shrink those fat cells and successfully reaching for the body you've always wanted.

The other thing you'll love about this plan is that it's designed to fit into *your* life, and it's a great economical way to get your body and mind in shape. I know your life is busy and that you can't afford to add another time-consuming activity to your to-do list. I totally understand. Because as a wife, mother, and working woman, my life is busy, too. Really busy. That's exactly how and why I came up with the Daily Dozen. You have to carve out some time for exercise, and everyone can find twelve minutes, your minimum daily requirement. You can get up twelve minutes earlier—which is what I like to do most of the time—or stay up twelve minutes later. You can shorten your gab-fest on the phone with a friend or get fit

WHAT YOU'LL NEED FOR YOUR DAILY DOZEN PLAN

- A pair of supportive sneakers.
- Two sets of weights—ideally one light and one heavy set.
- A mat or towel for floor exercises.

SHAKE THOSE SHIN SPLINTS

Arch muscles in our feet tend to deteriorate with age, making us more prone to shin splints. If you experience that tender pain along the shinbone when you walk or if you have a falling arch or flat feet, you can tone up your arches and calves with this towel-pull exercise. While in bare feet, sit in a chair and place a rolled-up towel just in front of your toes. Grab the towel between your toes and forefeet. Unroll it, flexing the arches of your feet as you do so. This prevents shin pain by developing your tibialis, arch, and shin muscles. Try it for a few minutes every other day for stronger, healthier legs and feet.

while watching your favorite TV show. However you squeeze in your twelve minutes, my point is that with my plan, you'll never have to make any kind of radical or jarring changes to your daily routine. It was created to make the most of every minute, because I know that every minute you have is precious to you.

My goal with the Daily Dozen and the minimum requirement of twelve minutes a day is to help you make exercise a daily habit. Just like brushing your teeth, I want exercise to become a natural, non-negotiable part of your life. I want it to be something that you pencil in your calendar daily and make a priority the way you would a doctor's appointment or business meeting. That's exactly what I do, and it works. When it's written in my calendar, it stays there and it gets done. I know you deserve to take at least twelve minutes a day for yourself to look and feel your best. I know you are worth it. My goal with these twelve minutes is to get you on track to a healthier life and to feeling better about yourself. Next month, you can work up to fifteen minutes a day, and eventually to thirty minutes, which is what I do. (Though on my busiest days I at *least* get my Daily Dozen in.) Try my Daily Dozen for twenty-one straight days and you'll be amazed at the changes you'll see and feel.

Benjamin Franklin said it takes twenty-one consecutive days of doing something to form a new habit. So why not form a healthy one? You can do it! It won't even take twenty-one days to see results. In fact, you'll see positive changes within the first week, whether it's looser clothes, more energy, or a better mood. And once you start, you'll see that this is a regimented, simple-to-follow plan that is guaranteed to help you lose weight. By the end of the first two weeks, you can lose up to twelve pounds.

In part 2, you'll see that each chapter corresponds to one day of the week. Simply open that chapter and you've got your exercise—and eating plan, which we'll get to in the next section—laid out for you in detail. It's that simple. You don't have to spend money for a gym membership or find someone to watch your kids. I don't want that stress in my life and don't want you to have to deal with it, either. I want to make exercise easy for you. This program can be done in the comfort of your own home on *your* schedule. It's also a plan that anyone can do. Don't be intimidated if it's been years since you've exercised. It doesn't matter whether you're a beginner or an expert. If you're trying to get back to your old weight or you're working to discover an all-new shapely body, you can do it! I can show you how! Exercise doesn't have to be difficult or monotonous. It can be fun.

Each day you'll do a twelve-minute workout that's very different from the day before.

- Monday: Cardio Fat Blast
- Tuesday: Lower-Body and Ab Workout
- Wednesday: Cardio Kickbox Workout
- Thursday: Upper-Body and Ab Workout
- Friday: Body Boot Camp Workout
- Saturday: Athletic Kettlebell-Inspired Workout
- Sunday: Yoga Stretch Workout

You'll also find a bonus workout just for your abs, a ballet-inspired barre routine, a few ways to tame tension at your desk at work, and exercises you can fit into the spare moments in your day that I call fidget-cisers.

They say that variety is the spice of life. It's true. Variety is also the key to why this plan works. It's why I know you'll get in the best shape of your life. By training this way—say, doing the Cardio Fat Blast one day, Lower-Body Workout another, and the Athletic Kettlebell-Inspired Workout the next—you're surprising your muscles and targeting them from different angles. You're also getting your heart rate up in new ways. This element of surprise and challenge is crucial in order for your body to change. Other-wise, if you work your body the same way every day, you hit a plateau and your body—and the scale—just won't budge.

The other easy aspect of the Daily Dozen is that it doesn't require lots of fancy, heavy equipment. All you need is two sets of weights (though many moves simply use your own body weight), a pair of supportive sneakers, and a mat or towel to do floor work on. That's it.

Speaking of weights, how do you decide which ones to choose? I suggest that you pay attention to your body's re-action to the repetitions you do for each exercise. I use five-pound and eight-pound dumbbells for most of the moves, but if you haven't been exercising for long, you can start at a lower weight and work up. Your body will tell you what you can lift. For example, when you're doing twelve repetitions of an exercise, the final two reps should feel tough. If they don't, the weight is too light—so add a couple of pounds. On the other hand, if you start to struggle long before the tenth repetition, it's too heavy. You'll need something a little lighter. Be sure to adjust the weights to accommodate your different muscles. Bigger muscles, such as those in your back, typically require heavier weights than smaller muscles like your triceps. It may take a little experimenting to see what works for you.

Though weights are important, what's *really* critical is that you maintain proper form and execute each exercise correctly. It's quality not quantity that is going to get you the fabulous results you want. You can do all the repetitions in the world, but if your form isn't correct you're not going to target the right mus-cles. Focus on good body alignment, on good technique, and on doing your very best. Give it all you've got for those twelve minutes! Make every second work for you. Take note of the special comments about form in each exercise, look at the photos, and aim to do each repetition as effectively as you can. Also, I want you to always improve, progress, and try harder to get to the next level. Thus some exercises offer a "challenge" option—an advanced way to do the move once you've mastered the basics. See which ones you can do—you may be surprised what your body can do if you just try. Remember, I am cheering you on! Success is within reach!

Your Weekly Dozen Miles

I'm a true believer that you need to do cardiovascular exercise (also called aerobic exercise) in order to burn fat and calories and change your body. That's why in addition to your twelve-minute Daily Dozen workouts, you need to do twelve miles of cardio exercise each week. This is a must. And it's the only way that you will lose up to twelve pounds in two weeks and drop a size—or two or three! The Daily Dozen exercises will boost your metabolism and tone you up. They'll sculpt and firm your muscles, but if you have a layer of fat covering up those muscles you're not going to see them.

The easiest cardiovascular exercise for most people is walking. All you need is a comfortable pair of walking shoes that have good arch support (to prevent feet from rolling inward) and that are flexible so they allow your feet to bend as you walk. And they should never pinch or rub even when they're new. If they do, they don't fit well.

I love to do interval walks to jump-start my metabolism and get a more effective workout in a shorter amount of time. An interval workout is where you intersperse fast-paced intervals of exercise with moderate paced intervals. For example, let's say that you typically walk at a pace of three and a half miles per hour for thirty minutes. If you mix things up and sprinkle in a few minutes of walking or running at, say, a five mph pace, you'll burn more calories in the same thirty-minute workout. Your heart rate rises when you're doing those fast-paced intervals, but it also stays up even when you switch to the slower-paced segments. And even if you aren't able right now to walk or run at five mph for an entire workout, you certainly can do it for a short period

GET AHEAD!

Keep your head in a neutral position for every exercise. To know what that feels like, stand with your back against a wall. Align your buttocks, shoulder blades, and head right up against the wall. Now walk forward. Take a moment to memorize that feeling.

AB-SOLUTELY NORMAL!

Don't get discouraged by ab work. It can feel tough, especially in the beginning. That's because short of getting out of bed, few movements in life mimic the abdominal crunch, so your abs really aren't challenged enough in an average day. In fact, they may well rank as the weakest muscles in your body. Just do your best. As a general rule, go until you start to feel the burn and then do two more. A few weeks of this and you, too, will have awesome, enviable abs.

of time, whether that's thirty seconds or several minutes. I want your ultimate goal to be doing a twelve-minute mile whether that's walking, power walking, running, or doing a mix of those things. In fact, I'm a member of the President's Council on Physical Fitness and Sports, which recognizes that the ability to walk/jog a twelve-minute mile is a sign of cardiovascular health. Make that your goal as you do your twelve miles of cardio each week.

One of my favorite metabolism-boosting walks is to mix two-, three-, and five-minute intervals. To determine the intensity of these intervals, think of your effort on a scale from 1 to 10, with 1 being a very easy stroll and 10 being so hard you can't carry on a conversation. You should never be at either of these extremes, but you should push yourself and be honest with yourself about how hard you're working.

1. 5 minutes: Warm up (intensity of 5).
2. 5 minutes: Walk at a moderate pace (intensity of 6).
3. 3 minutes: Power walk (intensity of 7).
4. 2 minutes: Walk at a moderate pace (intensity of 6).
5. 3 minutes: Speed walk (intensity of 8).
6. 2 minutes: Walk at a moderate pace (intensity of 6).
7. 3 minutes: Speed walk or jog (intensity of 9).
8. 2 minutes: Walk at a moderate pace (intensity of 6).
9. 5 minutes: Cool down at a moderate pace (intensity of 5).

You can mix things up by varying whether you walk on flat terrain or an incline, or whether you walk inside on a treadmill or outside on the open road. You can also carry a weight—just two pounds or lighter—in each hand to tone your upper-body muscles as you stroll. If you focus on breathing deeply and walking with good posture, you'll also be working your core muscles.

In addition to walking, there are so many other forms of cardio that can get you moving and count toward your twelve miles a week. This includes swimming, biking, the elliptical machine, and stair climbing. In any of these forms of activity, you can also do metabolism-boosting interval workouts to burn more calories and work harder in less time. Simply alternate one minute of faster-paced activity with four minutes at a slower pace. As you get stronger and more fit, increase the length of those fast-paced segments and scale back the slower-paced ones. As long as you're getting your heart rate up, it counts toward your twelve miles a week. You can do the same form of exercise for all twelve miles each week (for example, all walking) or mix it up doing a few miles of walking, a few miles of swimming, and a few miles of biking. You can also divide the miles any way you like. Perhaps one week, you want to do two miles a day for six days. Other weeks, you'll walk five miles twice a week and bike for two miles on another day. However you choose to do your twelve weekly miles, mixing and matching your cardio will keep each routine inspiring. And the results will be amazing!

> ## DON'T HOLD YOUR BREATH!
>
> It's important to keep breathing when you work out in order to bring oxygen to your muscles and give you energy. Try to match your breathing to your movement, and to breathe in through your nose and out through your mouth. Breathing also helps you relax, and it gives you renewed strength to execute your exercises and ready your body for whatever's coming up next.

Make Every Day More Active

In addition to your Daily Dozen workouts and twelve miles a week, I want you to be as active as possible on a daily basis. I really believe that one reason I've stayed in such good shape over the years isn't just because of regular exercise but because I keep moving. No matter where I am, I don't sit still for long, and I make the most of every moment. Recently I was on a flight from DC to Phoenix.

The winds were so bad that instead of five hours, the trip took nine, because we had to stop and refuel. Most of the other passengers just sat for the entire time, but not me. I was walking the aisle to get my circulation going and stretching in the back of the plane. And at home when I'm brushing my teeth, I'll do squats. When I'm waiting for my toast to pop up, I can squeeze in thirty push-ups leaning on the kitchen counter. Like I always say, your muscles don't know whether you're exercising in gym clothes during a formal workout or not. They just know you're working them. I don't just do this to tone up, I do it to boost circulation throughout the day: Circulation is what heals your body, and we all can use healing on a daily basis. I call some of these movements fidget-cisers (see Twelve Favorite Fidget-cisers on page 16), and I swear they keep me fit. They're one reason why I have more energy today than I did when I was twenty years old.

It's also easy to sneak in more walking during the day! Get off the subway a few stops earlier, park farther from the mall, and walk instead of drive to the coffee shop in the morning. Make yourself tiny promises: You'll circle the block twice before you buy your lunch; you'll take the stairs instead of the elevator whenever possible. If you want, purchase an inexpensive pedometer—it hooks onto your clothing and counts your steps for you.

The more you move, the more fit you'll be!

You should aim for ten thousand steps a day, but do the best you can! You'll be amazed at how quickly the steps add up. Just push yourself to increase your number each day and you'll get to your fabulous new shape—one step at a time!

Of course, looking great in your jeans isn't the only reason to do your Daily Dozen workouts and get fit. Getting in shape makes you healthier so you can do more and live longer. A recent study in the *British Journal of Sports Medicine* found that you can delay biological aging by ten or more years just by staying aerobically fit. Other research has shown that exercise can prevent an array of health risks from heart disease to cancer to osteoporosis. Working out will also help your soul and your spirit. It will improve your well-being and your energy level. It will change your life. You will feel recharged and energized. No more feeling sluggish or lethargic. No more tossing and turning at night. You'll sleep like a baby. And this feel-good effect is like a snowball. Once you see the benefits of just twelve minutes a day and eating well, you'll likely add other healthy habits to your life. You'll want to keep going because you'll see how wonderful you look and feel when you're living a healthier lifestyle. Just remember, there are three things in life that are all up to you: how *you* eat, how *you* move, and how *you* think. Eat healthy foods, move every day, and be optimistic. That's the basis of the Daily Dozen Plan and a very healthy, happy life. You can do it! I have faith in you!

Twelve Ways to Add Physical Activity to Your Daily Routine

Keeping up with your exercise sessions—a walk, a bike ride, a strength-training workout—is great and goes a long way toward burning calories and making you feel fit. But don't forget the importance of working more physical activity into your daily routine! One easy way to remind yourself is to think about every little step you take. This helps keep your body burning calories all day long. If you're sitting all day, your body isn't burning the calories it wants to. Sitting is the fastest way to gain weight—except for lying down. I'm a big believer in doing easy activities without getting sweaty. Short bursts of activity like that can really add up—which is what you want when you're trying to lose weight. Here are some tips on stepping your activity up a notch:

1. Dance your dinner off. Whether you're out on a Saturday night or staying at home, turn on your favorite tunes. The beat will keep you moving your feet, not to mention burning off some extra calories.

2. Stand up every hour on the hour and stretch your arms overhead. It opens your chest and brings oxygen into your lungs. It's great for circulation and enhancing your energy level.

3. Take the stairs instead of elevators. In addition to burning more calories, you'll save time—one study showed that waiting to ride an elevator takes twenty seconds longer than climbing up one flight of stairs. Today, see if you can take the stairs at least once when you normally wouldn't. Then tomorrow, do it twice. In no time, you'll be a stair master! If you need to go up several flights and can't climb them all, try a combination of the stairs and the elevator. Every step counts!

4. Walk up the escalator rather than just riding along. You'll burn calories and get to where you're going in no time.

5. Decrease your dependency on your car and see how many errands you can run (or how much commuting you can do) by bike. Biking is fantastic exercise because it helps tone your legs and gives you a great fat-blasting cardio workout.

6. If you live in a house with more than one level, bring things up or down the stairs as needed rather than letting a pile gather and *then* doing so.

7. If you're blessed with the gift of gab—as I am!—use that time to your fitness advantage. Instead of sitting on the couch or in a chair, pace back and forth.

8. Try this wall squat next time you're chatting on the phone. Stand up and lean your back lightly against a wall, making sure to press your spine flat. Then, as if you are sitting down in a chair, slowly lower your body along the wall until your knees are bent to at least a forty-five-degree angle (but don't go lower than ninety degrees). Hold the position for as long as you can. Start with twenty seconds and work your way up to sixty-second intervals. Repeat the exercise every few minutes during a phone call and you'll really give those thighs a workout!

9. At work, walk to a co-worker's office to tell him or her something rather than e-mailing. Not only will you burn a few calories and stretch your legs, but you'll reap the benefits of making a human connection instead of a computerized one.

10. Walk your kids to school rather than driving them. Childhood obesity is a huge epidemic, and physical education classes at many schools are being cut from school schedules. So if it's possible to walk to your child's school from your home, do so. You'll help establish healthy habits at a young age—and that's priceless.

11. Lift and lengthen your legs while you cook. I stretch my legs like a ballerina using my kitchen countertops. Just lift your leg, place your heel on the counter, and, with your abs in, fold over your leg and reach for your toes. Do this and other stretches often enough and you will be able to touch them one day.

12. After food shopping and loading your car with your groceries, walk your shopping cart back to the store instead of leaving it in the store's parking lot.

Twelve Favorite Fidget-cisers

While I aim for thirty minutes of official exercise a day, I never miss an opportunity to move. Your muscles don't know if you're in a fancy gym or the kitchen. This means that you can tone the 640 muscles of the body anytime, anywhere. You can turn idle time into toning time and do exercises and stretches while dinner is simmering on the stove or you're chatting on the phone. I call these one-minute exercises fidget-cisers, and I truly rely on them to help keep me trim and toned. Research has shown that little bursts of exercise throughout the day can increase your calorie burn up to a startling five hundred calories or more per day! Yes, five hundred calories! Here are twelve of my favorite anywhere-around-the-house fidget-cisers:

1. Sink 'n' Squat

Shape your butt in the comfort of your own kitchen!

▸ Stand about an arm-length away from the sink with your feet shoulder-width apart. Squat down and hold for 5 seconds.

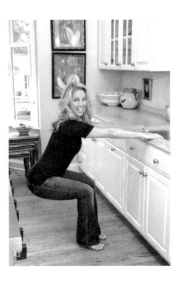

2. Leg and Butt Lift

You'll tone up and look fabulous from behind!

▸ While standing at the sink washing dishes or scrubbing veggies, lift your right leg up behind you and pulse it up and down. Switch legs and repeat.

3. Saddlebag Slimmers

Target this trouble spot in minutes.

▸ Stand with your left side to the counter and place your hand on it. Lift your right leg out to the side about a foot off the ground and pulse. Turn so that your right side faces the counter, then switch legs and repeat.

4. Inner-Thigh Toner

Lift the jiggle away.

▸ Stand with your left side to the counter and place your hand on it. Lift your right leg off the floor and bring it across the front of your body toward the left side. Pulse. Switch sides and repeat.

5. Telephone Thigh Trimmer
Get lean while you gab!

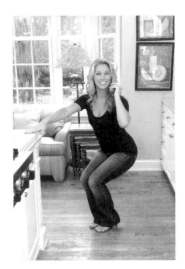

▶ While on the phone, stand about an arm-length away from a countertop. Place your right hand on the counter, hold the phone in your left, and bring your feet together. Squeeze your legs together as you squat down.

6. Countertop Push-Aways
I do these while waiting for my toast to pop up.

▶ Place your hands on the counter a little wider than shoulder-width and step a few feet away with your legs.

▶ Bend your elbows, bringing your chest toward the countertop, then push back up to the start position.

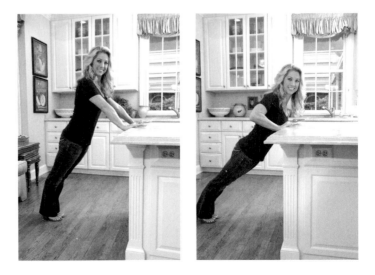

7. Down Dog

Squeeze a few of these in throughout the day and your back will thank you.

▸ Stand about two arm-lengths away from a countertop. Place your hands on the counter, bend forward at the waist so your body forms a ninety-degree angle, and keep your back straight.

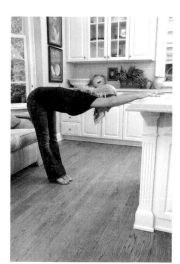

8. Leg Stretch

Another good move to do while you're waiting in the kitchen.

▸ Place your straight leg on a countertop. Keeping your back straight, lean forward, reaching for your toes.

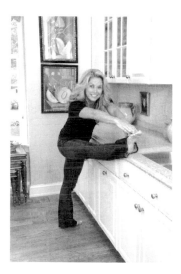

9. Couch Dips

Do these dips during commercial breaks and the backs of your arms will firm up fast.

▶ Sit at the edge of the couch. Place your palms on either side of your body and move forward so your body is off the couch. Bend your elbows behind you as you lower your body toward the floor. Keep your knees, thighs, and feet together with knees bent. Extend your arms to return to the start.

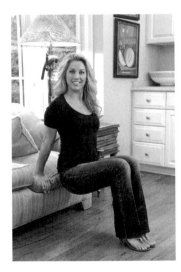 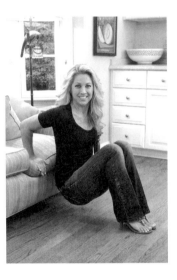

10. Tummy Tucks

Proof that you can tone your abs anywhere, anytime.

▶ Sit on the couch with your hands on either side of your body, palms on the couch, legs bent, and feet together and lifted off the floor. Using your abs, crunch your legs in toward your upper body.

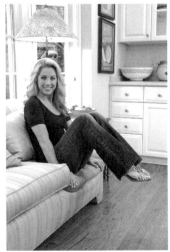

11. Lower-Tummy Toner
Flat abs for couch potatoes!

▸ Sit on the couch with your hands on either side of your body, palms on the couch, legs bent, and feet together with toes on the floor. Alternate lifting one leg at a time, gently tapping your toes on the floor.

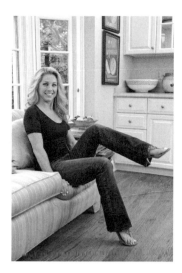

12. Back Relaxer
Unwind from a long day with this one.

▸ Sit on the couch with your legs together and feet flat on the floor. Lift your right leg up, place your hands just below your knee, and round your upper body forward. Switch legs and repeat.

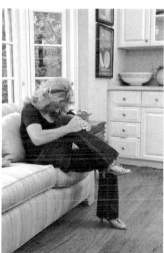

Food is fabulous, and having a good relationship with it will make you healthy and happy! You can do it!

The Daily Dozen Eating Plan

If you want to lose weight, drop a size, and get healthy while eating delicious, filling foods, then the Daily Dozen Eating Plan is your recipe for success. I love food and love to eat, but I also want to stay in the best shape possible. As a result, I've worked hard over the years to come up with a way to enjoy flavorful, satisfying meals and snacks that fuel my busy life yet keep me trim at the same time. The result is the Daily Dozen Twelve Foods to Eat Every Day. This is not a diet but a simple, lifelong way of eating that provides you with all the nutrients you need to stay healthy, slim down, and maintain your weight.

The word *diet* can have negative associations. It might make you think of that friend of yours who was desperately trying to lose weight for an upcoming class reunion. When the pounds didn't melt off quickly enough, she resorted to skipping meals (a definite no-no!) and working out until she reached the point of complete exhaustion. Not so appealing—or healthy, for that matter! But you can relax, because that's not what my program is all about. Changing the way you eat and incorporating healthy foods into your life doesn't have to be overwhelming. And that's exactly why my Daily Dozen Eating Plan comes down to a few simple principles that are easy to get the hang of. Trust me, you can do it!

It's called "chasing" a dream for a reason. Nobody gets anything by sitting still!

People often comment on my eating habits. They say that they can't figure out how I stay so fit when they see me eating all the time. Well, all that eating *is* my first secret. When you eat, your metabolism revs up and burns calories simply to digest your food. Munching at regular intervals throughout the day—rather than starving yourself or skipping meals—capitalizes on this metabolism boost by keeping that calorie burn running. My second secret for staying slim is the foods that I eat. Yes, *what* you choose to eat does make a difference not only in terms of keeping you full but also in providing the right nutrients to lose weight and stay healthy. And yet what's surprising to so many people is that there are tasty, filling foods you can enjoy while trying to shed pounds. You'll see that when you follow the Daily Dozen Eating Plan. (Think Yogurt Parfaits, Grilled Shrimp with Honey-Kissed Grilled Pineapple, Fish Tacos, and Chicken with Cilantro & Lime.)

The Power of Twelve

The basis of my eating plan is the Daily Dozen—twelve foods to eat every day. I don't mean twelve specific foods—like blueberries or chicken—but rather food categories. By having a varied, balanced diet of these twelve nutritious, wholesome, energizing foods, you can eat well and shed pounds and fat. I believe in whole foods with minimal processing. These twelve foods are:

1. Veggie
2. Veggie
3. Veggie
4. Fruit
5. Fruit
6. Fruit
7. Protein
8. Protein
9. Protein
10. Healthy grain
11. Healthy grain
12. Healthy fat

DAILY DOZEN SERVING SIZES

- *Fruit:* 1 medium-size whole fruit; 1 cup cut-up fruit or berries
- *Vegetables:* 1–2 cups
- *Protein:* 3–4 ounces meat, fish, or chicken; 1 cup dairy; ½ cup beans
- *Grains:* 1 slice bread; ½–1 cup grains, cereal, or beans
- *Healthy fats:* 1 teaspoon olive oil; a quarter of an avocado; 1–2 tablespoons natural peanut or almond butter; 2 tablespoons vinaigrette salad dressing; 1–2 tablespoons nuts

Yes, it's that simple. But eating three servings of vegetables, three servings of fruit, three servings of protein, two servings of healthy grains, and one serving of healthy fat for a total of twelve works. To create the menus in the Daily Dozen, I worked with registered dietitian and sports nutritionist Chris Mohr, PhD, a weight loss expert who has helped thousands of people lose weight permanently. Every single meal and snack is carefully created to help you finish your Daily Dozen and consists of the most wholesome, fresh foods you can find. You'll also find a checklist for each day of the Daily Dozen so you can monitor whether you're getting these twelve important foods. In order to make eating the Daily Dozen way a cinch, we have done all the homework and calculations for you! (To keep it simple and help you save time, I've also included a shopping list for each week at the end of the book.)

Chris and I designed unique menus that are a balance between the Daily Dozen Foods and a specific calorie count for each week. The latter is important because weight control comes down to one simple equation: calories eaten compared with calories burned. If you regularly eat more calories than you burn, you will gain weight. If you regularly burn more calories than you eat through work, play, and exercise, you'll lose weight. If you equalize the calories you burn and consume, you'll maintain your weight.

The goal of the first two weeks of the Daily Dozen Plan is to lose weight, so the meal plans for those days will be lower in calories. The first week, you'll eat around twelve hundred calories a day for women and fifteen hundred for men. The second week you'll eat around thirteen hundred calories a day for women and sixteen hundred for men, and add regular morning snacks. (Because men are typically larger than women, they need more calories.) Given the kinds of foods I've included, you'll actually feel totally satisfied regardless of the calorie count. No bird-size portions here! The goal of the third week is to help ease you into your new, healthy lifestyle while still shedding pounds. In that week, the Daily Dozen Meal Plans include fourteen hundred calories a day for women and seventeen hundred for men. For the first three weeks, I'd like you to stay as close to the Daily Dozen menus as you can: They're carefully formulated for you to lose

weight, and I want you to see results. I know these daily menus work (in conjunction with exercise, of course) because these are the same foods that I eat and have been eating for years. They'll also get you on the right track to eating healthfully and teach you how to make choices that are good for you.

The great thing about eating with the Daily Dozen Foods in mind is that you're focusing on the delicious, wholesome foods that you *should* eat, not lamenting a long list of foods that shouldn't pass your lips. As a result, you don't feel deprived, but rather that you've got a lot of edible options. This positive way of thinking is another reason I love this plan. When it comes to all areas of life, I believe that looking at the bright side and having a glass-half-full attitude can make all the difference in terms of how successful and happy you are. And that goes for your diet, too.

In the next sections, we'll cover each of the wholesome, fresh Daily Dozen Foods including their serving sizes and why they're so important for a healthy mind and body—as well as looking great in your jeans. You'll find lists to give you an idea of where different types of food fit into the Daily Dozen. Some foods even do double duty—like nuts, which are listed as both protein and healthy fat. I've focused on foods that are most commonly available, but feel free to expand beyond these lists and add things like star fruit or hearts of palm, which can give an attractive and exotic flair to your usual salad. There's a whole world of healthy food out there to explore!

Fruits and Vegetables

Produce is one of the most important things that you can eat when you're trying to lose weight. Because fruits and vegetables contain a lot of fiber and water, they fill you up for very few calories. The result? You can eat more of them while still losing weight. Proof comes from a *Consumer Reports* survey of 32,213 people who were trying to shed pounds. About 70 percent said that eating vegetables and fruits helped them lose weight and keep it off. The other good thing about fruits and vegetables is that there are so many to choose from and so many healthy ways to prepare them.

*All the exercise tips in the world won't work unless *you* work. Get moving!*

Though the Daily Dozen Plan calls for eating three servings of vegetables a day, eating more than this is okay since vegetables are so low in calories and so high in fiber and water. Most veggies have ten to fifteen calories per serving. Even the few exceptions—such as avocado, lima beans, and potatoes—are just around a hundred calories per serving. Best of all, they keep you feeling full, and they're vitamin-packed.

When it comes to fruits, you can eat more than three servings, but not as much as you want. Unlike vegetables, fruits typically contain more natural sugar—and as a result more calories. One easy way to get your fill of fruits and vegetables is at breakfast. Simply mix berries or sliced fruit into your cereal or yogurt or add at least three different types of vegetables to an omelet. (One of my favorite combinations is onions, tomatoes, and mushrooms.)

Besides keeping you satisfied, fruits and vegetables are bursting with many important nutrients like vitamins, minerals, and antioxidants, which are compounds believed to help reduce your risk of many diseases and age-related illnesses. A produce-packed diet is a crucial part of a healthy lifestyle. The science that supports this is amazing. For example, cabbage contains vitamins C and B as well as disease-fighting compounds called indoles that are believed to boost your body's own cancer-fighting enzymes and possibly halt the cancer process once it's begun. Research suggests that broccoli may be the richest source of sulforaphane, another compound that stimulates the body to make more cancer-zapping enzymes. Plus, just one cup has six grams of fiber (which is crucial for weight loss), the entire daily recommended level of vitamin C, and 25 percent of the recommended levels of vitamin A and folate. Two other favorite veggies of mine are kale and spinach, which studies show are brimming with powerful antioxidants called lutein and zeaxanthin. These compounds help protect your eyes from cataracts and macular degeneration—the leading cause of blindness. Spinach and kale are also rich in folate, a B vitamin that helps prevent birth defects during pregnancy, lowers blood levels of homocysteine, and may protect against colon cancer and heart disease. As you'll see, many of my Daily Dozen recipes and meal plans contain these super foods.

When it comes to fruits, tomatoes are a real powerhouse. (Yes, they're fruits not veggies, but I grouped them under veggies as well since that's how most of us think of them.) Studies show that lycopene, the nutrient that gives tomatoes their beautiful red color, may cut cancer risks in half for people who regularly consume tomatoes and tomato products. Eating raw tomatoes is tasty and good for you, but there are even more nutrients in tomatoes when you roast or cook them because the heating process helps release them. Other amazing fruits are berries, which are chock-full of healthful compounds and fiber, too! Blueberries are one of the best sources of antioxidants compared with other fruits and, along with cranberries, help stave off urinary tract infections. Strawberries pack a big nutritional punch since just a cup provides nearly double your daily vitamin C requirement and also contains a potent anticancer agent called ellagic acid. And fruit in general may ward off the bone-thinning disease osteoporosis, according to a British study, which found that women who ate the most fruit as children had denser, stronger bones.

On a more beautiful note, eating vegetables and fruit will help you look your best, giving your skin and hair a healthy

DIVIDE AND CONQUER

If you're eating too much candy at work and overeating in the evening, pick only one of these problems to tackle at a time. Then give yourself weeks to move on to the next issue. You'll feel overwhelmed if you try to tackle too much at once. Also, since problems are often related, you'll be surprised that solving one may get rid of the other.

glow. For example, blueberries are full of antioxidants that reduce wrinkle-causing inflammation, while sweet potatoes contain vitamin C, a nutrient that boosts collagen production.

When it comes to produce, your goal each day should be to have a rainbow of colors. That's because the foods in each group offer you different essential nutrients that you need to feel and look your healthiest. The reason I designed the Daily Dozen Plan as I have is so that you hit these different groups with every meal. For example, on one Daily Dozen Meal Plan you may have red bell peppers in your scrambled eggs for breakfast, a spinach salad for lunch, and some glazed carrots with dinner. Obviously this balance of color can't happen all the time since some days you may not have a certain food in the house, but it should be your goal.

Your Daily Dozen Vegetables

DAILY DOZEN SERVING SIZE: 1–2 cups of vegetables

GREEN VEGETABLES
artichokes
arugula
asparagus
avocado
basil
bok choy
broccoli
broccoli rabe
brussels sprouts
celery
chives
cilantro
collard greens
cucumbers
dandelion greens
dill

green bell peppers
kale
leeks
lettuce (romaine, red leaf, Boston, and
    Bibb are the best)
lima beans
okra
parsley
snap green beans
snow peas
spinach
string beans
Swiss chard
tomatoes
turnip greens
watercress
zucchini

RED/PURPLE VEGETABLES	YELLOW/ORANGE/BEIGE VEGETABLES
beets	butternut squash
eggplant	carrots
radicchio	corn
radishes	mushrooms
red bell peppers	onions
red cabbage	orange bell peppers
red chard	potatoes
rhubarb	pumpkin
	sweet potatoes/yams
	yellow bell peppers
	yellow squash

I know that there are certain fruits we tend to eat over and over again because they're top of mind. But it's important to mix things up and aim to get your Daily Dozen requirement of fruit from different types of these naturally sweet treats. I tend to think of fruits in three categories, and if you get one from each you'll do a good job getting the mix of nutrients you need to slim down and stave off an array of diseases. First there are the easy-to-grab fruits that fit into the palm of your hand, require no more preparation than a quick rinse, and can be found almost anywhere. They're a quick way to get antioxidants on the run. The second group is the tropical and citrus fruits, which offer you different nutrients than the easy-to-grab variety and that you need to peel and cut up. And then

A TERRIFIC TIME SAVER

Pre-planning meals will help free up time to exercise during your week. To avoid dinnertime chaos, I use Sunday as my meal-planning day. I prepare what I can for the week ahead, pick out recipes, tally up ingredients, grocery shop, and pre-chop what's necessary. Sometimes I broil or grill chicken so I can use it later in the week in salad or fajitas. This way I don't have to take time out each day (and away from exercise) for last-minute preparations.

there are the tiny fruits like berries that are a huge help when you're trying to lose weight and improve your health. Again, you'll see that the Daily Dozen Meal Plans are carefully thought out to include fruits from each of these groups so you reap an array of benefits. Even the squeeze of lemon in the recipes is going to help you!

Your Daily Dozen Fruits

DAILY DOZEN SERVING SIZE: 1 medium-size piece of fruit or 1 cup cut-up fruit

EASY-TO-GRAB FRUITS
apples
apricots
bananas
grapes
nectarines
peaches
pears
plums

TROPICAL AND CITRUS FRUITS
grapefruit
kiwi
kumquats
lemons
melons
oranges

papayas
passion fruit
pineapples
tangerines
tomatoes
watermelon

TINY FRUITS/BERRIES
acai berries
blackberries
blueberries
cherries
cranberries
pomegranates
raspberries
strawberries

Protein

Protein—the word comes from a Greek word meaning "of prime importance," and it is critical for weight loss, since it helps you build and repair muscle and keeps you feeling full longer. There are three important categories of protein, and if you can get all three into your day—or aim for it—you're doing great!

Plant sources of protein are a menu must if you're a vegetarian. However, what most people don't realize is that they're important for those of us who eat meat, too, and their benefits go beyond the waistline. According to a huge government survey of more than ninety-six hundred Americans, people who eat beans four times a week are 22 percent less likely to get heart disease than people who eat beans less than once a week. Beans also lower blood cholesterol level and blood sugar and are full of iron and B vitamins. Another non-animal protein source is soy foods. They can be prepared in many delicious ways and have been linked to the prevention of osteoporosis, lower cholesterol levels, a reduced cancer risk, and even a reduction in menopausal

EATING ON THE GO

Stash good-for-you emergency snacks like raw almonds, dried fruit, and whole-grain breakfast cereal in your purse. Or do what I do and hard-boil a dozen eggs on Sunday. I slip two at a time in little plastic bags and store them in the fridge to eat on the run. Cutting up fruits and veggies works the same way. All these things protect you from the temptation of the vending machine or convenience store snacks.

symptoms such as hot flashes. Soy sausage, patties, hot dogs, and ground veggie round are great substitutes for beef or pork. Miso, a grainy paste made from soybeans, is an excellent ingredient for marinades, sauces, and soup bases. For a quick nutritious pick-me-up, try soy nuts, roasted soybeans, or a bowl of steamed edamame.

I limit my red meat intake to about once or twice a month and instead try to eat fish more often. But if you choose red meat, look for the leanest cuts and grass-fed meat; otherwise they can contain too much artery-clogging saturated fat. Beef eye round and top round, flank steak, pork tenderloin, lamb foreshank, and veal leg are excellent choices with no more than 25 to 30 percent of calories from fat. For any other cuts of meat, simply trim off any visible fat and pay attention to your portion size. Use skinless chicken and turkey to cut down on fat without cutting meat out. I often use ground turkey breast instead of ground beef to make spaghetti sauce, tacos, and sloppy joes, and swap savory chicken sausages for those made with pork.

Calcium-rich dairy foods like skim or low-fat yogurt, milk, and cheese are another good source of protein. Of course, you probably know that calcium-rich foods keep your bones strong and prevent osteoporosis, but they may also help you slim down—that is, if you choose the lowest-fat versions. Research reveals that people who get the recommended daily allowance (one thousand milligrams for those under the age of fifty and twelve hundred milligrams for those over fifty) lose more weight than people who get less calcium. Unfortunately, about 75 percent of American women don't meet this requirement, according to the US Department of Agriculture. Though there are calcium-rich options for every meal of the day, breakfast is a great time to fill your diet with calcium: In addition to dairy foods, you can enjoy fortified breakfast cereals and juices.

Your Daily Dozen Proteins

DAILY DOZEN SERVING SIZE: 3–4 ounces of meat, fish, or chicken; 1 cup of dairy; ½ cup of beans/barley/lentils, etc.

PLANT SOURCES OF PROTEIN
almond butter
barley
beans
chickpeas
hummus
lentils
natural peanut butter
nuts
peas
quinoa
soybeans
tofu

FISH AND LEAN MEAT
chicken
duck
eggs
halibut

lamb
lean ground beef, turkey, or pork
mahi mahi (dorado)
pork
salmon
shellfish
steak
tilapia
tuna (fresh or canned in water)
turkey
veal

LOW-FAT DAIRY PRODUCTS
cheese
cottage cheese
cream cheese
skim milk
sour cream
yogurt

Healthy Grains

Whole grains are a diet essential because they help fill you up thanks to all the fiber they contain. Fiber works by turning on the "burn fat" signal in your body and acting as a multitasking marvel that fills you up, so you don't fill out! Very simply, fiber takes up a lot of room in your stomach—think of it like a dry sponge that has been soaked in water—meaning fewer hunger pangs! It also lowers insulin levels. The hormone insulin is the blood glucose cleanup crew. When blood glucose rises after eating a high-carbohydrate meal, insulin rushes in, scooping up this glucose and depositing it in cells for use as energy. But if you can't use it for immediate energy, it gets stored as fat. Thus you want to keep those glucose levels as stable as possible; fiber helps you do just that. In two different studies, fiber-champion cereals—oatmeal and bran—squared off against cornflakes, which are virtually fiber-free. After eating the high-fiber cereals, people were able to make it to lunch without feeling hungry. Those who started with cornflakes listened to their stomachs growl. Go fiber! This is why you'll love the healthy grains I combined in the 4 Minute Grains cereal that you'll have for breakfast a few days.

It's important to know that there are actually two types of fiber. Soluble fiber is found in oats, barley, apples, pears, edamame and other soy products, dried beans and peas, and fruits. This type of fiber may reduce your risk of heart disease by mopping up artery-clogging cholesterol, and help prevent diabetes by regulating your glucose levels. Insoluble fiber is found in wheat bran, whole wheat products, and most vegetables. This type of fiber may alleviate constipation by helping wastes move through your system faster.

Your Daily Dozen Healthy Grains

DAILY DOZEN SERVING SIZE: 1 slice of bread, pita, tortilla, English muffin; $\frac{1}{2}$–1 cup of cooked grains or pasta, cereal, or beans

GRAINS
barley
brown rice
buckwheat
bulgur

cereals made from healthy whole grain
    (such as Wheatina)
couscous
millet
oatmeal

popcorn
quinoa
wild rice

HEALTHY BREADS, ETC.
crackers
pasta
pita

rye and pumpernickel bread
spelt bread
sprout bread
tortillas
whole-grain English muffins
whole-grain waffles
whole wheat bread

A Dozen Tips from Denise: Simple Tips for Filling Your Life with Fiber

Fiber is super important for slimming down and sticking with your healthy eating goals. It's also pretty easy to add more fiber to your life. You'll be amazed how a few simple substitutions can help increase how much fiber you get in your diet and how full you feel. Try these tips and you'll feel healthier and fabulous in no time!

1. Swap cornflakes (zero grams of fiber in one ounce) for a bran-based cereal (five to fifteen grams).

2. Instead of white bread, which has just one gram of fiber per slice, switch to whole wheat bread, which has two to three grams.

3. Leave white rice and pasta behind and go for brown rice or whole wheat pasta. Some people think whole wheat pasta isn't as tasty as white; experiment with different brands to find one you like.

4. Fill a whole wheat tortilla (which has five grams of fiber compared with one or two in the white flour variety) with steamed veggies for a yummy, low-cal wrap.

5. Eat fruit with breakfast every morning. Try berries with your cereal, slice a banana into yogurt, or add diced apples to oatmeal while it cooks.

6. At lunchtime, bulk up your sandwiches by adding lettuce, tomatoes, and onions, and have a small salad or cut vegetables on the side.

7. Throw a bag of mixed frozen veggies in the microwave for a veggie side dish that's ready in minutes! Add vegetables to casseroles, soups, rice dishes, and baked goods—almost anything is better with more vegetables!

8. Eat your beans. Throw half a cup (eight grams) of drained red kidney beans in your salads or in your chili to perk it up.

9. Drink plenty of water as you work on increasing your fiber intake. At first you may feel bloated, and water helps move things along.

10. Eat cut-up vegetables with hummus as a snack. Just one tablespoon has a gram and a half of fiber and 12 percent of your daily calcium needs. Plus it has compounds that fight heart disease and cancer

11. Remember that high-fiber carbs, like apples and oatmeal, are "good carbs" that'll help you lose weight. Enjoy these fiber-full foods whenever possible!

12. When reading food labels, look for those that have at least three grams of fiber per serving.

Healthy Fat

Though the word *fat* makes most people cringe, it's actually an important part of your diet and a source of fat-soluble vitamins—A, D, E, and K. It will help you lose weight. The key is to make sure you're eating the right kind. Good fat helps slow your stomach from emptying so you feel full longer. Healthy fats are those that are unsaturated such as monounsaturated and polyunsaturated fats, which are believed to reduce your cholesterol and have other health benefits. These good fats can be found in olive oil, nuts, avocados, flaxseed, other plant foods, and fish. Omega-3 fatty acids are also a good fat and are believed to reduce inflammation throughout the body. Studies suggest that omega-3 fatty acids can reduce the risk of heart disease, stroke, and Alzheimer's and prevent arthritis pain. These healthy fats are also credited with helping to alleviate depression, allergies, and asthma—even with keeping hair looking and feeling soft and silky. Though you can find this nutrient in avocados and olive oil, it's plentiful in fattier fish like salmon, herring, lake trout, sturgeon, bluefish, anchovies, and sardines. There's also a plant form of omega-3 fatty acids called alpha-linolenic acid, which you can find in flaxseed and flax oil, canola oil, and soybean oil. Like fish oils, this fat has also proven to be heart-healthy.

The "bad fats" that you should avoid include saturated fats, the artery-clogging fat found in fatty meats, chicken skin, whole milk, cream, regular cheese, and butter. While it's okay to have a little of this fat, too much raises blood cholesterol and promotes heart disease. Another bad fat is trans fat, which is found in the partially hydrogenated oils used in regular margarine and many processed foods. Trans fats may be even worse than saturated fats. While both raise blood levels of artery-clogging LDL cholesterol, only trans fat lowers levels of beneficial HDL cholesterol. I know it's hard if you're used to eating fatty foods, but once you replace them with the healthy stuff, you'll hardly miss them!

Your Daily Dozen Healthy Fats

DAILY DOZEN SERVING SIZE: 1 teaspoon of olive oil or flaxseed oil, 2 tablespoons of avocado, 1 ounce or 2 tablespoons of nuts, 1–2 tablespoons of natural peanut butter

SOURCES OF UNSATURATED FATS
AND OMEGA-3 FATTY ACIDS
almond butter
avocado
canola oil
flaxseed
flaxseed oil
grapeseed oil
herring
mackerel
natural peanut butter
nuts
olive oil
salmon
seeds
sunflower oil
vinaigrette salad dressing (healthy oil
 and vinegar)

Water

Drinking water is a critical part of losing weight. Water doesn't contain any calories, but it helps make you feel full. (Try sipping a glass right before meals to help you eat less.) Aim for at least eight 8-ounce glasses a day, because your cells cannot metabolize excess fat without water, and your organs cannot eliminate toxins without this miracle drink. Your body also needs water for digestion,

FRUIT SWAPS

You'll be eating a lot of yummy, healthy fruit on the Daily Dozen Plan. But just in case one meal or snack's fruit suggestion doesn't work for you, you can swap it for one of the following. In other words, they're all interchangeable. This way you still get your Daily Dozen Foods and stay within the right calorie count. You can even mix them up, if you like—for example, by having half a cup of raspberries and half a cup of blueberries, or a plum and a tangerine.

half a grapefruit	1 apple
1 orange	1 cup raspberries
1 cup pineapple	1 cup blueberries
1 peach	1 cup blackberries
2 plums	1 pear
1 cup sliced kiwi	1 cup cherries
1 medium banana	2 nectarines
1 cup chopped melon	1 cup sliced mango
1 cup strawberries	2 tangerines
1 cup grapes	

temperature regulation, and much more. I always drink two glasses of room-temperature water when I get up in the morning. After sleeping for seven to eight hours, your body is dehydrated and craves water. I also suggest you drink a glass with each meal and snack and every fifteen to twenty minutes during a workout so that you'll have more energy to finish your session (or even exercise longer than you planned!). Make it easy to access water by installing a filter in your water tank or on your kitchen faucet. I just did and it's great. I fill up my reusable food-grade stainless-steel bottle so I always have a refreshing drink at hand. I mention stainless steel because though more research needs to be done, some experts believe plastic water bottles contain chemicals that may be harmful to our health. To play it safe, I've opted for stainless steel over plastic. It's good for my family and the environment.

YOUR DAILY DOZEN REQUIREMENT: Eight 8-ounce glasses of water

*   *   *

Now that you know more about the Daily Dozen Eating Plan, it's time to get started. Just note that at this point, your eating is going to be quite structured, and as I mentioned earlier, I want you to stick closely to the menus for each day. All Daily Dozen Meal Plan recipes are for one serving. This is not only to help you lose weight, but also to make this whole plan super easy. Just a note if you're going out to dinner during these three weeks: Try to order something similar to what's on the plan. For example, if the Daily Dozen dinner is grilled salmon, then order a nice piece of fish and ask them to go easy on the oil and hold the butter.

Once you hit the weight you want to be, you will probably do what I do and keep a mental tab based on making sure you get the twelve important foods for the day. For example, midmorning I usually follow up breakfast with a fruit snack of banana, apple, orange, half a grapefruit, or berries. At lunch I remember to squeeze in more veggies by eating a spinach salad, making an arugula, tomato, and turkey sandwich, or having vegetable soup. (Soup takes time to eat, which helps slow you down and prevents you from overeating!) At dinner, I try to eat two more vegetables such as steamed broccoli and asparagus. I've even included recipes for some of my favorite twelve-minute meals at the end of the book—proving that healthy food for the whole family doesn't need to take a lot of time. But no matter how busy I am, as long as I get those daily dozen, I know I've eaten well that day.

Another important point I want to make is that the Daily Dozen Meal Plan really mixes things up so that you never get bored. That's another one of my secrets. I have a lot of variety in my diet. One day I'll eat oatmeal with flaxseed for breakfast; the next, I'll have a Yogurt Parfait. I love to eat fruit for snacks—some days I'll have half a banana with a handful of blueberries; other days, sliced kiwi. The same goes for lunch or dinner. I love eating salads but I don't stick to the same old, same old lettuce. One day the basis of my salad is spinach, another it's some red, leafy greens. As you can see, there's a lot to choose from.

Now that you know the basics, you're ready to get started. Remember that you can do whatever you set your mind to. You are worth the time and the effort. I can't wait for you to be the fit and fabulous person you want to be—and you *will* be! Be positive about the road ahead of you. The results will be well worth it! You can and will succeed!

GO ORGANIC?

While no research proves yet that organic foods are nutritionally better for you, there are several good reasons to buy organic. For one, such foods are wholesome—and better for the environment! Foods labeled USDA Certified Organic are grown without the use of pesticides, synthetic fertilizers, or genetically modified organisms, and organic meats and dairy products are free of antibiotics and growth hormones. Choosing organic foods also supports local farmers who use renewable resources and promote soil and water conservation. The downside to buying organic is that because it costs farmers more to produce these foods, they're often more expensive than their conventional counterparts. That's changing as more and more stores offer these products, but you may want to be selective about which organic foods you buy. I know that I am.

When it comes to produce, whether I go organic or not depends on the specific fruit or vegetable. For fruits that aren't as easy to wash, I buy organic. One example of this is berries, because I simply don't have the time (or desire) to sit and scrub each little berry. If it's a bigger fruit or vegetable that's easier to clean or one with a thick skin like oranges, avocados, or bananas, I'll go for what's on sale but don't feel that buying organic is a must. The Environmental Working Group, a nonprofit, has put together a list of foods that it calls the Dirty Dozen because they typically have the most pesticides. They are:

1. Peaches
2. Apples
3. Bell peppers
4. Celery
5. Nectarines
6. Strawberries
7. Cherries
8. Kale
9. Lettuce
10. Grapes (imported)
11. Carrots
12. Pears

When it comes to other foods like meat or dairy, I'll definitely go organic if I'm buying something that has fat in it, because the fat is where chemicals tend to accumulate. When it comes to fat-free dairy products, I sometimes buy what's on sale. But whether or not you go organic, the most important thing is that your food choices are healthy ones!

Half a Dozen Tension Tamers

These are quick simple moves that you can squeeze in throughout your day to de-stress and relax your body. I do them when I'm at the computer because I know that a muscle will stay in a state of tension unless there is a change of activity. Circulation is what helps heal your body. These tension tamers only take a few minutes and can be done without even getting up from your chair. I'd suggest holding each pose for at least twelve seconds. Do them regularly and you'll be amazed at how good you feel.

1. Reach Up

This helps lengthen the spine and give space to each vertebra.

▸ While sitting in a chair, extend your arms toward the ceiling. Reach up as you lengthen your back.

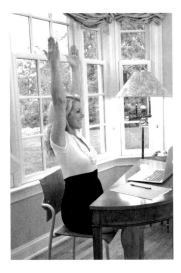

2. Back and Side Stretch

Alleviate back tension in one sitting.

▶ From a seated position, place your right hand on your chair and lift your left arm up overhead. Stretch and lean your body over to the right. Repeat for the left side.

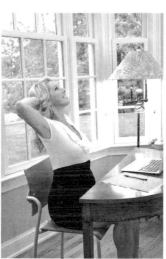

3. Chest Lift

Improve your posture by doing this daily. Better posture makes you look slimmer.

▶ Sitting up straight in a chair, bend your elbows and place your hands behind your head. Lean back, open your chest, and look up toward the ceiling.

4. Wrist and Forearm

A must for preventing wrist pain or, even worse, carpal tunnel syndrome.

▸ Sitting up straight, extend your left arm out at chest height with the palm facing up. Use your right hand to put pressure on the left fingers and stretch the palm forward. Then use your right hand to gently press your fingers down toward your body. Switch hands and repeat.

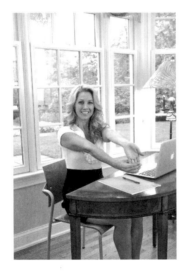 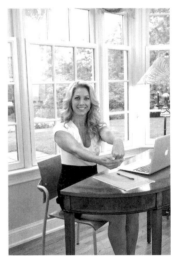

5. Waist Twist

This cures a multitude of aches, from your back to your shoulders.

▸ Sitting up tall, twist your body to the right and place both hands on the back of your chair or armrest. Use your hands to help twist your upper body to the right even more. Switch sides and repeat.

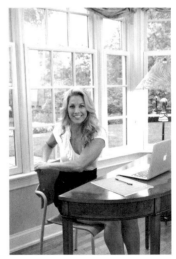

6. Neck and Shoulder Relaxer
Do this anywhere to release tension.

▸ Sitting up tall, bend your elbows and place your hands behind your head. Gently press your head forward and feel a stretch along the back of the neck.

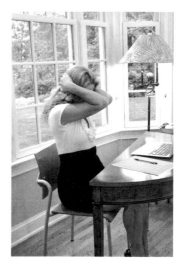

Frequently Asked Questions

Q: I see that the Daily Dozen Plan starts on a Monday. But what if I start reading your book on a Thursday or other day of the week?

A: First of all, congratulations on picking up this book and taking the first step to a healthier, better-looking body. I believe that there's no time like the present to get started, so I don't want you to wait another minute to do so. Instead, open the book to the day of the week you're on—in this case, Thursday—and follow the week one workout and eating plan for that day. Continue doing this until Monday comes. At that point, start with Monday's week one workout and eating plan and follow along from there. This way you've simply given yourself a few bonus days to get fit and eat right. The results will be worth it. I promise!

Q: Can I drink alcohol on the Daily Dozen Plan?

A: I love a good glass of red wine once in a while myself. Not only because it tastes good but also because it's got lots of phytonutrients and potent antioxidants like resveratrol, which are good for your heart. However, for the first week of the Daily Dozen plan, you shouldn't have any alcohol and should stick closely to the food plans for each day. This helps you clean out your body and get on the right track. In week two, you can add a glass of wine if you'd like. Just skip your morning or afternoon snack and save those calories for a glass of wine in the evening. But only *one* drink, because drinking your calories away isn't as filling as eating them. Also, alcohol tends to lower your inhibitions; if you drink too much, you may also find yourself eating too much or eating the wrong foods.

Q: **Can I drink coffee and tea on the Daily Dozen Plan?**

A: Again, it's all things in moderation. Tea is fine and calorie-free as long as you don't load it up with lots of milk and sugar or use artificial sweeteners, which studies have shown can actually make you gain weight. In fact, I love tea with lemon in the late afternoon when a craving strikes or as something soothing (decaf) to sip before bed. Green tea is fabulous because it's loaded with nutrients, and research suggests that it has amazing health benefits. That said, any kind of tea can be a satisfying treat, and there are so many flavors from fruity to spicy that your options are endless. I actually go in seasons and have a soothing cup of hot tea when it's cold out and a refreshing glass of iced tea in warmer months. If you like coffee, you can have one cup a day. Just make sure to limit what you put in it because, again, calories from milk, sugar, and creamers can add up quickly. I have one cup of coffee in the morning and just add a splash of skim milk. And definitely steer clear of those calorie-rich drinks available at most coffee bars. These drinks are more like a dessert. All that syrup, whipped cream, and sugar means some of them weigh in at an astonishing four to five hundred calories, or more!

Q: **What do I do if I am allergic to or don't like one of the foods on the plan? For example, one day you have fish, and I can't stand fish.**

A: Naturally, you shouldn't eat anything that will adversely affect your health. I also believe food is something you should enjoy, so I'd be the last person to tell you to eat something you didn't like just to lose weight. If the plan calls for something you can't eat or just can't stand, simply replace that meal with another meal that's similar. For example, if it's a protein-based dinner of fish that you don't like, look for a dinner within the same week that's also protein-based, like a chicken or bean dish. This way you're probably getting the same items from your Daily Dozen Food list and keeping the calories close to where they should be for that week.

Q: **After years of being inactive, I'm trying your Daily Dozen Plan. After a short time, I'm hooked! But how do I get my family moving, too?**

A: Congratulations! Realizing the importance of exercise is one thing, but actually making the commitment to get fit—and healthy—is truly commendable! And it's fantastic that you'd like to encourage your family to exercise as well! Don't worry, getting your family fit shouldn't require begging or bribes. Here are some ideas:

■ Check out my fitness DVDs that everyone can do together. You can even pick out something that taps into their interests. For example, if your husband is a golfer, he might like a sport-specific DVD that features stretches and workouts that'll help improve his swing. Or maybe my *Best Belly Fat-Blaster*s DVD that my husband uses. And if your daughter likes to dance, there are plenty of kids' DVDs she can try.

■ Turn on your kids' favorite radio station or make a mix of tunes with a good beat and turn your living room into a disco.

■ Engage in some friendly competition. Go to the park and see who can speed walk or run the fastest from point A to point B, or play a game of volleyball at the beach or pool.

■ Go biking together, throw around a Frisbee in the backyard, or go ice-skating. As long as the activity's fun, getting everyone moving will be a snap!

Q: **Should I take vitamin supplements on the Daily Dozen Plan?**

A: We should all try to get all our vitamins from the food we eat; that's what my meal plan is all about. But because it can be hard to eat perfectly every day and to be sure I get the full amount of all the vitamins I need, I take supplements as my little "insurance." Personally, I like Nature Made vitamins, and this is what I take every day: a multivitamin, a vitamin C (500 mg), a vitamin D (1,000 IU), calcium (1,200 mg), and fish oil (1,200 mg). But check with your doctor to find out what your own specific needs are.

Q: I cook for my spouse and kids, not just myself. Is it okay for my kids to eat the foods on the Daily Dozen Plan?

A: Definitely! In fact, my kids and husband have been eating these meals for years. Though one goal of the Daily Dozen is to help you lose up to twelve pounds in two weeks, the other goal is to teach you how to eat healthy foods. That's why every single meal on the plan is nutrient-rich. Even if your spouse and kids don't need to slim down, we *all* need to get as many vitamins, antioxidants, and other important nutrients as we can. By cooking this way for your kids, you'll get them on the right track to healthy eating and teach them how delicious good-for-you foods actually are. This is critical considering our country is experiencing an unprecedented epidemic of childhood obesity. They'll enjoy these tasty meals so much, they won't even know they're eating healthy food. And who says you have to tell them?

Q: I have a young child. How did you find time to work out when your children were babies?

A: I admit, it wasn't always easy! When Kelly and Katie were in diapers, it was all about tending to their needs. But I still never let a day go by without trying to fit in some activity! I'd put them in their strollers and take long walks, carry them (believe me, your arms will get toned!), or squeeze in my regular workouts during their naptime. Where there's a will, there's a way! You can do the same, especially because the Daily Dozen workouts are designed for a busy life like yours. Just do the minimum daily requirement of twelve minutes while your child is napping or strap her into her bouncy seat or high chair and let her watch you. (You'll be amazed at how entertaining it is to see Mom or Dad breaking a sweat!) Keeping exercise a priority when your kids are small is a smart thing to do. You'll be happier and less stressed, which will help you be a much more positive and energetic parent. And you'll teach your child that fitness is a natural part of daily life, just like brushing your teeth. Everyone wins!

Q: **I work very late hours and rarely have time to cook. I know that eating out all the time isn't healthy, but it's so much more convenient to pick up pizza, Chinese, or burgers. What other options do I have?**

A: The good news? You have plenty of options. It sounds like you'd benefit from preparing meals ahead of time and then storing them in the fridge or freezer. That way, all you have to do when you get home is reheat the food. I do this a lot on Sundays, and it really saves time and makes my busy week easier. At the grocery store, always look for quick-prep side items. For example, plain frozen veggies can be steamed in the microwave in less than ten minutes, as can instant brown rice. You can also pick up some prepared foods from the deli counter, such as roasted turkey and rotisserie chicken (just avoid the fatty skin of the poultry, as well as mayo-laden pasta and potato salads and coleslaw). When eating take-out is truly unavoidable (try not to let this happen more than once a week), go for healthier options, like steamed shrimp and vegetables (with sauce on the side) from your local Chinese restaurant, a grilled chicken sandwich or a single-patty hamburger minus the cheese from the neighborhood burger joint, or a grilled steak with lots of veggies or chicken fajitas (without fatty extras like sour cream) from the nearby Mexican chain. Enjoy!

Q: **I tend to be an emotional eater—someone who heads to the refrigerator when I'm stressed, upset, even happy. What can I do to curb this kind of eating?**

A: First of all, you're not the only one who dives into a bag of chips or a pint of ice cream when times get tough. Almost all of us are emotional eaters at least sometimes (including me!). Sometimes we turn to food to ease emotion or celebrate, such as when we feel happy, sad, anxious, or excited, even though we're not hungry. And the foods we turn to are usually comfort foods that are high in calories and fat and low in nutrients, like ice cream, cookies, and chips.

Emotional eating is nothing to be embarrassed about, but if you allow yourself to eat emotionally on a regular basis, it can be harder to follow a healthy diet and maintain a healthy weight. And I know that's not what you want. You can control emotional eating. You just need another outlet for your emotions so you don't continue to use food to calm down or help yourself feel better. One of the best ways to do this is by keeping a journal. Writing down what's going on in your life and the challenges you are struggling with provides that emotional release you're seeking, so you don't need food for comfort. Take some time to think about exactly what you're feeling, and choose the right words, so they truly represent your emotions. You can put them down on paper or on your computer—your choice. Write at least one journal entry a week, although more is always better! You'll come to love writing in your journal and see it as a secret friend. I know I do!

Q: How can I overcome nighttime snacking? I know I'm eating because it's a habit and I'm bored, but I can't stop.

A: This is one of the most common questions that I get. One way to curb this late-night eating is to make sure you have an afternoon snack, which can stabilize you for your entire evening. It helps keep your metabolism going and curbs your appetite before you go home so you don't go nuts. Another way I keep myself from overdoing it at night is by putting a curfew on the kitchen. After 8 PM, turn off the lights and tell yourself, "The kitchen is closed." If you have a door, close it and mentally note that the room is off limits. Another trick is to brush your teeth as soon as you hit that curfew and even rinse with one of those minty mouthwashes. Trust me, nothing—not even your favorite tempting treat—tastes good when you've got that minty taste in your mouth.

Q: What's the best way to track my weight loss? Is it weighing myself or measurements?

A: I actually think both the scale and a tape measure are great ways to monitor your progress. The scale is good to keep you on track, but it's not perfect.

First, water retention can cause fluctuations in weight (up to four pounds). And because muscle weighs more than fat, the scale may not budge while your body is getting smaller and you're losing inches. In that case and because muscle takes up less room than fat, a measuring tape will show you how well you're progressing. Though you can weigh yourself weekly on this plan, take your measurements on day one and then wait until day twenty-one to take them again. You'll see the inches just melt off.

Use a flexible tape measure to find out the circumference of your waist, hips, thighs, chest, and upper arms and write down all the numbers (don't worry, this is for your eyes only!). Here's how:

■ **Waist:** Although it may be tempting, try not to suck in your belly when you're measuring your waist. Take a deep breath, let it out, and then measure wherever is smallest. If your waist seems to be all the same size, measure around your belly button.

■ **Hips:** Measure at the very biggest part.

■ **Thighs:** Measure wherever they are the biggest. Make sure to measure both thighs.

■ **Chest:** Measure all the way around your chest and back right at your nipple line. For women, make sure not to squish your breasts as you measure.

■ **Upper arms:** Measure around the biggest point above your elbow. Make sure to measure both upper arms.

■ **Vertical buttocks length:** This is the distance from the top of your rear to the bottom of each butt cheek (where a pair of traditional underwear would end). You may be able to twist your body around and take this measurement yourself, but it's better if you can enlist someone else to do it from behind (no pun intended!). This is less scientific than some of the other measurements, but it's fun to see the change in your cheeks. My girlfriend did the Daily Dozen workouts for three weeks and found that her rear lifted two inches!

	DAY 1	DAY 21
WAIST		
HIPS		
RIGHT THIGH		
LEFT THIGH		
CHEST		
UPPER RIGHT ARM		
UPPER LEFT ARM		
RIGHT VERTICAL BUTTOCK		
LEFT VERTICAL BUTTOCK		

Q: Can I eat chocolate or any other sweets on this plan?

A: I like dessert, too, and am definitely not willing to banish it from my diet. After all, life is too short, and sometimes I just need a piece of chocolate! Plus, you probably know that cutting one whole food group out of your life just sets you up to crave that food and binge on it in days to come. The way I fit sweets into my life is to eat a little less of something else that day. For example, if I want to have some chocolate after dinner, I'll skip my afternoon snack. Do the same on the Daily Dozen Plan and you'll easily be able to squeeze in some treats. But don't have dessert during week one, and remember when you do substitute in later weeks to do it rarely—desserts might be delicious, but they don't give you a full feeling or lasting energy.

Q: Can you recommend anything to help boost my energy levels?

A: There's no shortage of things you can do to create more energy! But first I'd look at your sleeping habits—people often need more energy because they regularly get by on less than seven hours of sleep. That's not enough! Although exercise, a healthy diet, and lots of water will definitely help energize you, nothing can compensate for a lack of sleep. So try to go to bed at the same time every night and get up at the same time every morning. And try to get a full eight hours of uninterrupted sleep!

Twelve Easy, Effective Ab Exercises

My tummy is flat and firm, and my secret is consistency. Working the abs and back at least three times a week or a few minutes each day—particularly after the age of forty—is the key to keeping them fit. And the great thing about the ab muscles is that they respond quickly to toning no matter your age.

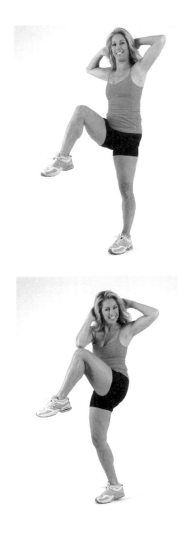

1. Warm Up
Get those stomach muscles warmed up to work!

▶ KNEE-UPS: Stand up straight with your abs pulled in tight and feet hip-width apart. Bend your elbows and place your hands behind your head. Alternate lifting your knees up to your chest. Time: 30 seconds.

▶ Continue alternating lifting your knees, but bring your opposite elbow to the opposite knee. Time: 30 seconds.

2. Waist Twist

Lose an inch—or two—around your waist!

▸ Holding a weight or two vertically in both hands, stand with your feet wider than hip-width apart, knees slightly bent, and toes pointed out.

▸ Keep your upper body upright. Hold the weights in front of your chest, contract your abs and twist from side to side, really rotating your upper body. Time: 1 minute.

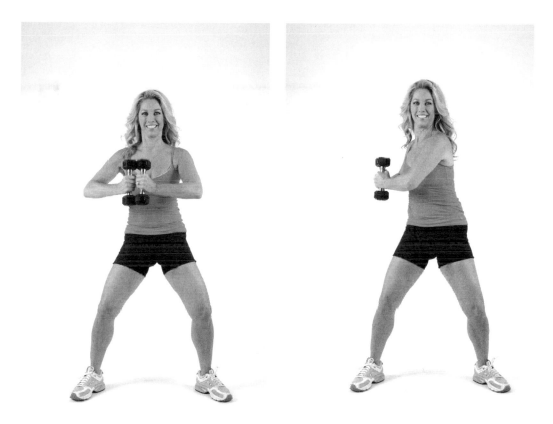

3. Ab Pull-Down
This works similar to the ab machines at the gym.

▸ Stand straight with your legs together. Hold a weight in each hand and bend your elbows so your hands are by the sides of your head.

▸ Bend your right leg as you lift it off the floor and bring your elbows toward your knee. Then do the same with the right knee. Continue to alternate. Time: 1 minute.

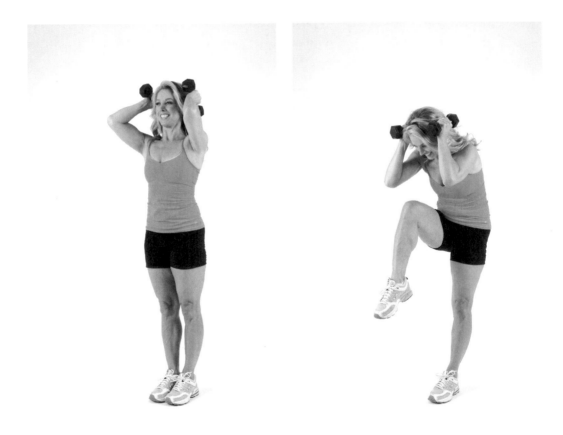

4. Weighted Roll-Ups
Tone your abs from top to bottom.

▶ Lie on the floor with your legs bent and just your heels on the floor. Hold one weight in both hands and extend your arms straight above your head.

▶ Lift your arms so they're extended straight in front of you as you engage your abs and roll your head, neck, and shoulders off the floor.

▶ Continue to roll all the way up until you're sitting up straight and extend your arms up above your head toward the ceiling. As you come up, really elongate the spine and stretch it up. Roll back down one vertebra at a time using your abs. Time: 1 minute.

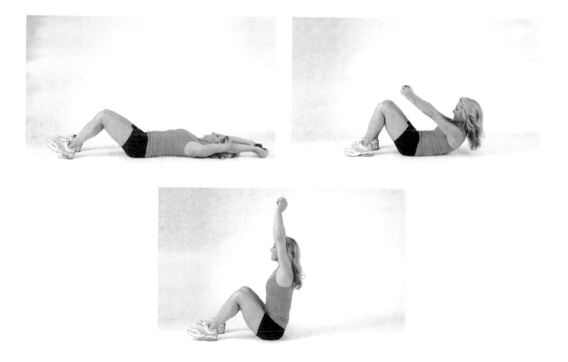

▸ Lie on the floor with your right leg bent and the foot on the floor, and your left leg bent so your left calf is under your right knee. Hold a dumbbell in your right hand and extend your arm straight above your chest. Place your left arm on the floor next to you.

▸ Roll up to a seated position, keeping the dumbbell extended toward the ceiling.

▸ Using your abs, lift yourself all the way up to standing with the dumbbell still reaching toward the ceiling. Then roll yourself back down to starting position. Time: 30 seconds. Switch sides and repeat.

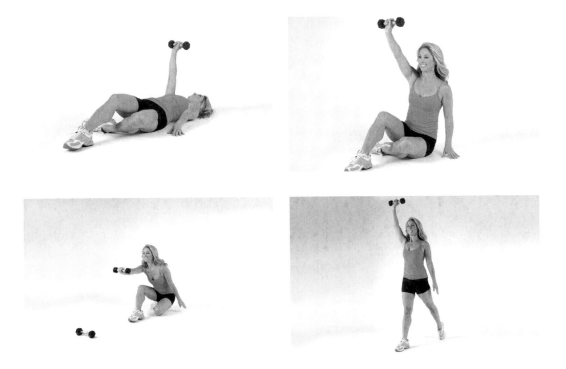

5. Oblique Toners

Twist your way to an hourglass waistline.

▶ Lie on your back with your legs bent and your feet flat on the floor. Tighten your abs and lift your upper body so that the shoulder blades are off the floor. Hold a dumbbell with both hands and bend your elbows so your hands are in front of your chest.

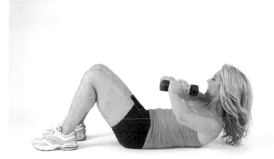

▶ Twist your upper body to the left side as you pull your abs in. Really feel the rotation as you crunch and twist to the side. Time: 30 seconds. Switch sides and repeat.

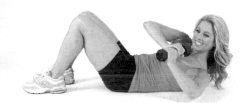

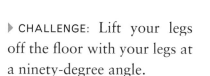

▶ CHALLENGE: Lift your legs off the floor with your legs at a ninety-degree angle.

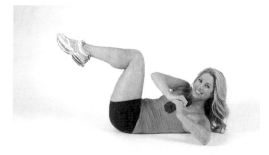

6. Lower-Tummy Toner

This targets the lower abs as well as the thighs!

▸ Lie on your back with your legs bent in the air at a ninety-degree angle and put a rolled-up hand towel between your knees. Place your arms by your sides with your palms on the floor.

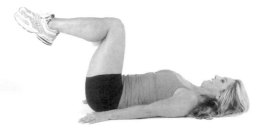

▸ Lift your hips up off the ground. Pull your belly button in and press your inner thighs together. Use your abs—not momentum—to lift your hips. Time: 1 minute.

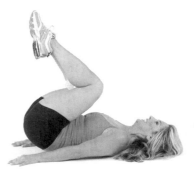

▸ CHALLENGE: Straighten your legs as you lift your hips off the ground.

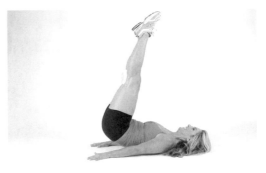

7. Double Crunch

I love this because it's a "complete" ab workout.

▸ Lie on your back with your legs bent at a ninety-degree angle in the air with a rolled-up hand towel between your knees. Bend your elbows and place your hands behind your head.

▸ Bring your lower and upper body in toward each other and crunch. Make sure you're pulling in your abs. Time: 1 minute.

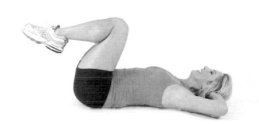

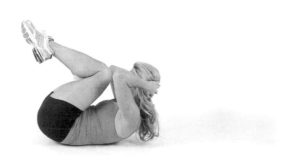

8. Knee Twists

This one is great for carving out a trim and slim waistline!

▸ Lie on your back with your legs bent at a ninety-degree angle off the floor, and place a rolled-up towel between your knees. Extend your arms out to the sides on the floor.

▸ Keeping your legs together, lower your knees to the left side. At the same time, keep your upper body still and your abs engaged.

▸ Switch sides bringing your knees to the right side. Alternate sides repeatedly. Time: 1 minute.

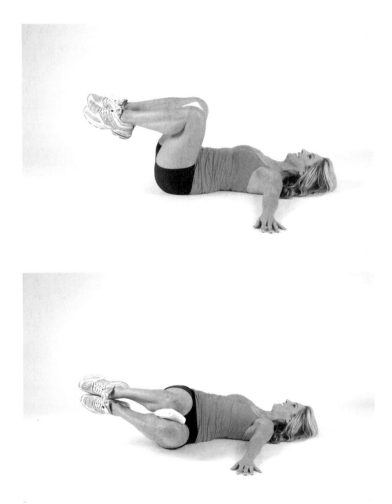

9. Flutters

Blast flab from your abs and inner thighs in one move. A total core exercise.

▸ Lie on your back with your legs extended straight up toward the ceiling. Place your arms by your sides, with your hands underneath your buttocks—this will really work your lower abs. Point your toes.

▸ Lift your head and shoulders off the floor, and alternate crossing your legs in front and back of each other, progressing to a forty-five-degree angle. Then slowly crisscross back up to start position. Time: 1 minute.

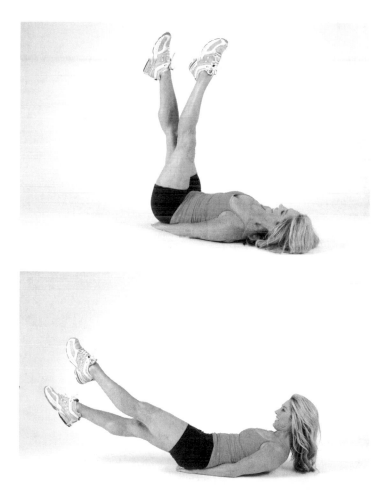

10. Plank Pull-Ins

This move zeros in on the transverse abdominis muscle, the one that keeps your tummy tight. Keep your body straight from head to toe!

▸ Position your body in a plank, balancing on your toes and palms. Keep your abs pulled in, back straight, and head extended so that your body forms one long line from the top of your head to your heels.

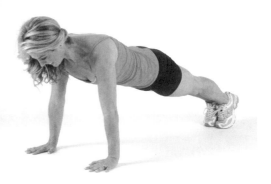

▸ Bend your right leg, bringing the knee toward your chest. Straighten the leg and bring your left knee toward the chest. Continue alternating. Time: 1 minute.

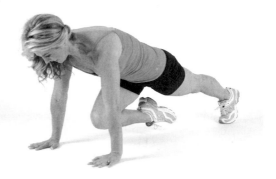

▸ CHALLENGE: Bring the knee to the opposite side of the body.

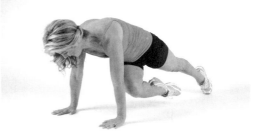

11. Upper Back Extensions

Strengthen your back muscles that line your spine and prevent injuries.

▶ Position yourself on your hands and knees. Extend your left arm out to shoulder height. At the same time, extend your right leg straight out behind you. Alternate arms and legs. Time: 30 seconds.

▶ Lie with your stomach on the floor, legs extended straight out behind you, and arms extended overhead.

▶ Look to your left side as you extend the left arm back behind you and the right arm out to the right side. Time: 15 seconds. Switch sides and repeat.

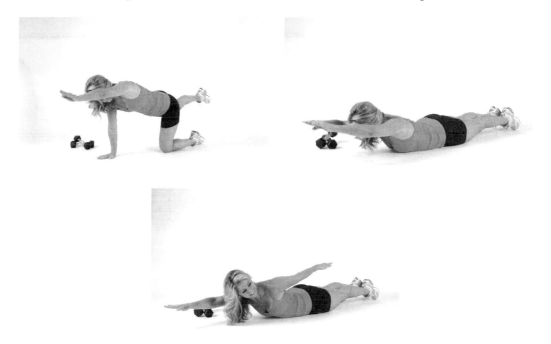

▶ CHALLENGE: Add light weights.

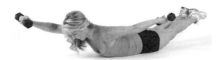

12. Cool Down
Stretching feels so good . . .

▸ Sit up straight with your legs crossed in front of you. Place your right hand on the ground and extend your left arm toward the ceiling. Lean over to the right side. Time: 15 seconds.

▸ From the above position, round the back forward and extend your left arm toward the right. Time: 15 seconds. Switch sides and repeat both stretches.

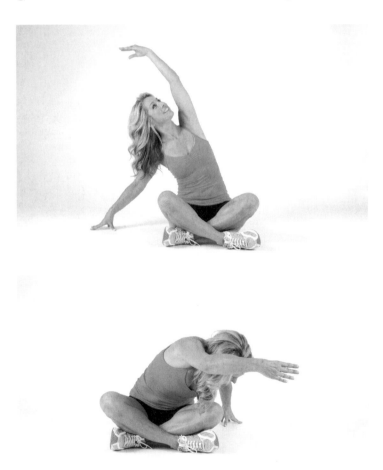

PART TWO

THE PLAN

If fitness came in a bottle, everyone would have a great body.
We will make simple lifestyle changes that really work!

Monday

Welcome to your Monday Daily Dozen workout! You've made the first step toward a fitter, healthier body and I know that you *can* do it. Simply stick with this plan, which I've designed to blend easily into your life, and you *can* change your body. You *can* get in the best shape of your life and have success. Just stay upbeat and positive. This is your time to shine. Go for it! And get excited for what lies ahead. You deserve to feel your best!

Today's Daily Dozen workout is twelve minutes of aerobic moves that I call the Cardio Fat Blast. As the name implies, it'll burn calories and fat, and jump-start your metabolism by mixing periods of moderate-intensity exercise with periods of higher intensity. Called interval training, this boosts your heart rate and challenges your body more than maintaining one steady speed would. This Cardio Fat Blast workout will also help tone your body with compound moves that require you to use a lot of muscles at one time. The benefit is that you're training like an athlete and working twice as many muscles in half the time! Remember, burning fat and calories is important, but so is building muscle. That's because muscle requires more calories to maintain

POSITIVE THOUGHTS

Do your exercise routine without judgment. Don't think negative thoughts like *I'm too fat* or *I'll never get this*. Simply trying will help you improve those push-ups and that chest fly. Replace judgment words like *lazy, weakling,* or *fat* with positive words such as *courage, challenge,* and even the phrase *I can*. Congratulate yourself on starting something new. You're amazing.

than fat. As a result, the more muscles you have, the more calories you burn even when you're *not* working out—and that includes sleeping and sitting on the couch.

This Cardio Fat Blast will do more than help you lose pounds and inches over the next three weeks; it'll also give you more energy in just twelve minutes! In fact, many fans of my *Daily Dozen* DVDs say they do this Cardio Fat Blast on other days of the week when they need an energy boost rather than seek out an unhealthy, short-term solution like sugar or caffeine. Trust me. I need energy for my long, busy days and, boy, does this workout help. So, let's get started on the road to the healthier, more fit you! I know you can do it, and more importantly, I want *you* to believe that you can!

MONDAY'S CARDIO FAT BLAST

Commit to being fit! You can do it! You are worth it!
Double the workout in half the time!

1. Punches

Warm up your body and tone your arms, all while revving up your metabolism.

▶ Stand with your feet wider than hip-width apart and pivot to your left side so that your left knee is bent slightly and your right leg is straight behind you. At the same time, bend your left arm so it's by your side with your fist by your shoulder and punch your right arm out to the left side at shoulder height. Then pivot your body to the right side and repeat. Alternate punching from side to side. Time: 20 seconds.

▶ Continue pivoting from side to side but now alternate punching your arms up straight toward the ceiling. As you punch your left arm up, lean to the right, bending the right knee slightly. As you punch with your right arm, lean to the left, bending your left knee slightly. Time: 20 seconds.

▶ From the above position, alternate punching your arms down toward the ground. Time: 20 seconds.

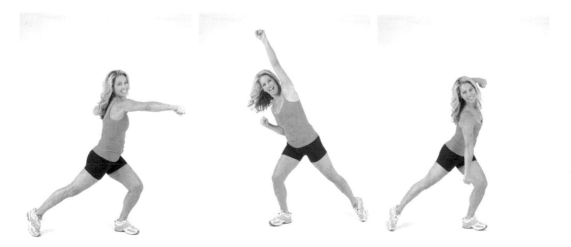

2. Knee-Ups with Abs
Trim your waist and slim your thighs. And get your heart rate up, too!

▸ Stand up straight with your abs pulled in and feet hip-width apart. Bend your arms so your elbows are out to the side and your hands are in front of your chest. Alternate lifting your knees up to your chest. Time: 20 seconds.

▸ Continue alternating lifting your knees, but place your hands behind your head with your elbows bent. This targets the front of the torso and lower abs, too. Time: 20 seconds.

▸ Continue alternating knee lifts, but bring your right elbow to your left knee and then your left elbow to your right knee. This targets the sides of the waistline. Time: 20 seconds.

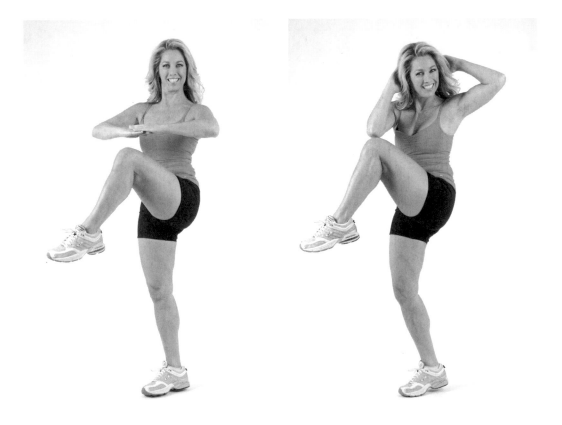

3. Power Jog with Arm Firmer
Just feel the fat blasting off your entire body.
Kick-start your metabolism into high gear.

▶ Jog in place, keeping your abs in tight and your back straight as you extend your arms down by your thighs with your palms facing away from you.

▶ BICEP CURLS: Pump and curl your hands toward your shoulders. Time: 20 seconds.

▶ TRICEP TONERS: Continue jogging in place, but now press your arms behind you. Time: 20 seconds.

▶ OVERHEAD PRESSES: Continue jogging, but change your arm movements so that you press up toward the ceiling between each bicep curl. Time: 20 seconds.

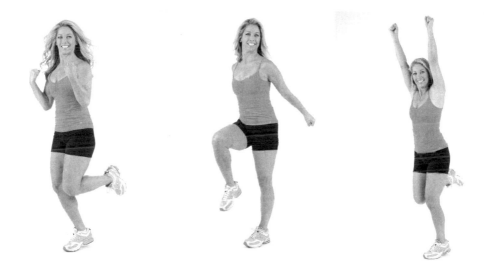

SUCK IT UP!

Did you know that the deepest layer of your abdomen is called the transverse abdominal? This muscle helps you contract your abdomen and draw your belly inward. So suck it up. Seriously. Repeatedly pulling in and tightening your abs will help create a natural girdle for the front of your midsection. It also adds power and stability to everyday movements such as walking and sitting.

4. Side Leaps/Lateral Bounding

Sculpt and shape your buttocks. And train like an athlete.

▸ Stand with your feet hip-width apart. Bend your knees and squat down. Bend your elbows with your hands up by your chest. From the squat position, step side-to-side about two to three feet. Time: 30 seconds.

▸ Keep moving side-to-side in a squat position, but leap from side to side rather than stepping and lift your foot up slightly off the floor. Time: 30 seconds.

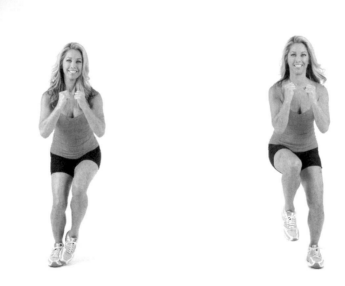

▸ CHALLENGE: While leaping side-to-side, swing your arms forward and back as you move.

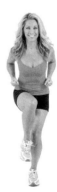

5. Hamstring Curl

Sleek, sculpted, sexy legs can be yours as you get heart-healthy, too.

▸ Stand with your feet wider than shoulder-width apart and place your hands on your hips.

▸ Step side-to-side about two to three feet as you alternate lifting one leg off the floor behind you and bringing your heel to your rear each time. Time: 30 seconds.

▸ BACK ROWS: Continue hamstring curls with your legs and add an arm variation where you're pulling your elbows down and back behind you. Time: 30 seconds.

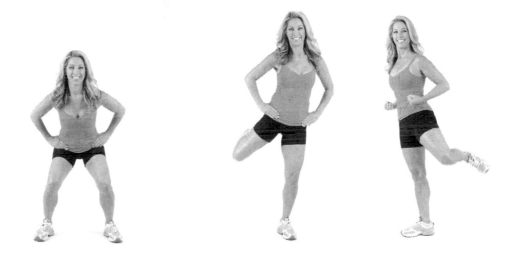

6. Burpee (Squat Thrust)

This is a tough one, but it works it all.
And it blasts calories fast to shrink those fat cells.

▶ Stand with your feet more than hip-width apart and squat down, touching the floor with your hands.

▶ Jump your body back with knees bent and abs strong.

▶ Jump your feet back toward your hands to the first position.

▶ Stand up and extend your arms toward the ceiling. Time: 1 minute.

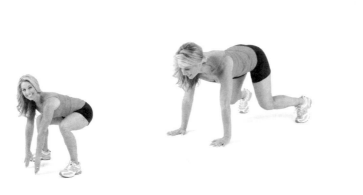

▶ CHALLENGE: When you jump your legs out behind you, straighten your legs as in the top part of a push-up/plank. Then add another challenge at the top: Jump up.

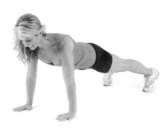

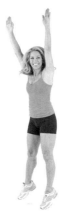

7. High Kicks

Kick your way to "hot legs." And get fit for life.

▶ Stand with your feet shoulder-width apart and alternate kicking your legs out in front of you (straighten them but don't lock your knees). As you kick, reach the opposite arm straight out in front of you at chest height. Time: 30 seconds.

▶ Continue kicking and reaching while twisting the upper body toward the leg that's kicking. Time: 30 seconds.

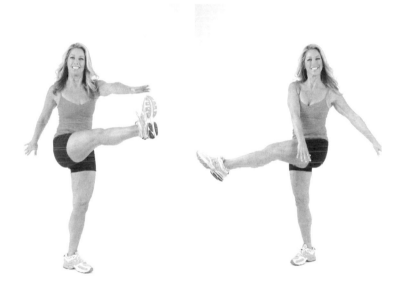

▶ CHALLENGE: Add some power to the move by jumping a bit off the floor each time you kick.

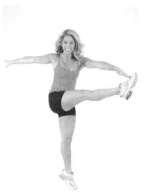

8. Step Butt Lift
Your rear end is the last thing people see when you leave the room.
Make it look great! Keep it up; this is where it counts.

▸ Place your hands on your hips, turn to your left, take a step forward with your right leg, and then extend your left leg straight behind you. As you extend your leg, extend your arms straight up toward the ceiling.

▸ Then repeat for the other side by taking a step back with your left foot and turning your body to the right as you step forward with your right foot. Extend your right leg straight behind you and your arms up toward the ceiling. Time: 1 minute.

▸ CHALLENGE: Repeat the same step but add power by jumping off the floor as you step to each side and extend the leg behind you.

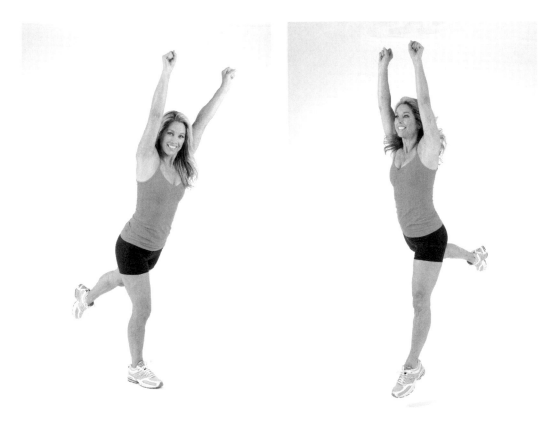

9. Twisters

Twist off fat and calories. And lose an inch around your belt.

▸ Here you're doing the twist! Stand with your feet shoulder-width apart and arms extended out to the sides at shoulder height. As you twist your legs to the left, swing your arms to the right; as you twist your legs to the right, swing your arms to the left. Time: 30 seconds.

▸ Bring your legs together and continue doing the twist, squatting down low for several twists and twisting back to standing. Time: 30 seconds.

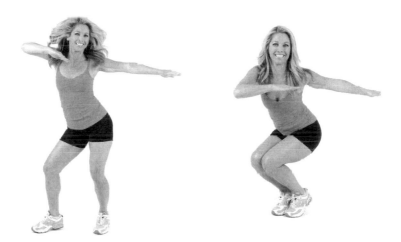

STOP SMOKING!

You'll prevent more than just lung cancer! While smoking is believed to cause almost 90 percent of all lung cancer deaths, it may also be involved in cancers of the throat, esophagus, larynx (voice box), kidneys, pancreas, stomach, cervix, and bladder. Plus, if you stop smoking, you'll stop exposing those around you—including your family—to harmful secondhand smoke.

10. Knee Lunge Series

You can't find a better move for toning and lifting your rear than the lunge.

▸ Stand with your feet shoulder-width apart and hands on your hips. Lift your left knee up to hip height and then step it behind you as you bend your right knee into a lunge position. Make sure that your front knee is at a ninety-degree angle and does not go over your toes. Time: Repeat lunges for 30 seconds with the left leg; then do 30 seconds with the right leg.

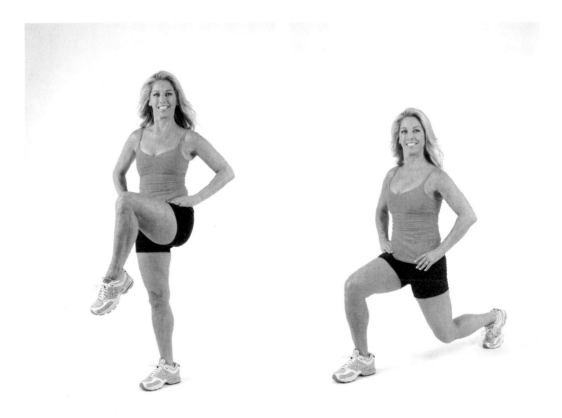

11. Standing Ab Toner

Focus on your core while you gradually bring your heart rate back down.

▸ Stand with your feet shoulder-width apart and then step your left leg behind you and bend into a lunge. Bend your arms by your sides.

▸ Pump your arms as you quickly lift your left leg on and off the floor using your abs and bring the knee to hip height. Time: 30 seconds. Then switch legs and repeat for 30 seconds with the right leg.

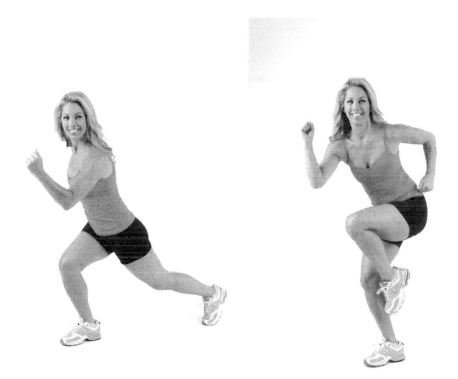

12. Cool Down

Reward your muscles for their hard work with these soothing stretches.
You deserve it!

▶ BACK STRETCH: Stand with your feet wider than hip-width apart and knees slightly bent. Place your hands on your thighs. Round your back, pull your navel in toward your spine, and feel the stretch in your back. Time: 10 seconds.

▶ CALF AND HAMSTRING: Bend from the hips and shift your weight onto your left foot and extend the right leg straight in front of you with the right heel on the ground and toes pointing up to the ceiling. Place your hands on your thighs and sit back slightly. Time: 10 seconds. Switch legs and repeat.

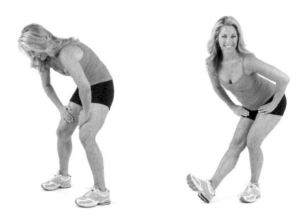

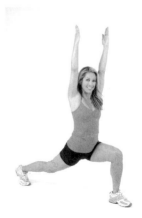

▶ EXALTED WARRIOR: Stand in a lunge position with your left leg in front. Make sure your left knee doesn't go over your left toes and straighten your right leg behind you. Keeping your abs in tight, extend your arms straight up toward the ceiling. Time: 10 seconds. Switch legs and repeat.

A Dozen Tips from Denise:
Boost Your Motivation to Eat Right and Exercise

Though the best way to get motivated is to see amazing changes in your body, your energy level, how well you sleep, and how well your clothes fit, there are times when your motivation may be lagging. When that happens, try these simple but effective tips. They always work for me.

1. Music is key to getting motivated, so I blast it when I work out. Upload songs to your iPod or treat yourself to a favorite CD, but only allow yourself to listen to your new music when you work out. It'll give you something to look forward to.

2. Give yourself a nonfood reward after a week's worth of healthy eating and exercise. Some suggestions: half an hour when you turn off the phone and curl up with a good book or magazine, getting a manicure, or buying yourself flowers.

3. Find a workout buddy. This *really* helps me stick with and look forward to my workouts. Every Sunday, I pull out my calendar and call my friends to set up exercise dates for the week. I love that I can stay in shape *and* stay in touch with friends—my BFF workout.

4. Make healthy living a cinch. Put your workout clothes out the night before or keep your gym bag stocked and in your car. These things make it easier to exercise, and just the sight of your workout clothes is a great reminder.

5. Hang a calendar somewhere that you can see it often—the refrigerator, above your computer   and put a sticker or special mark on the days you work out and eat right. Seeing evidence of your hard work will inspire you to keep it up.

6. Pick a time of day that you're going to exercise and stick with it. This way it becomes part of your schedule and makes you feel more committed. It's like an oath to yourself that you won't want to break. For example, I know that Monday, Wednesday, and Friday, I'm going to exercise at six thirty with my husband before taking our kids to school, and Tuesday and Thursday, I'll do it after I drop them off. Without some planning, your day can easily get ahead of you.

7. Pick a close friend and e-mail your workout log to him or her each week. When you know someone else is "watching," you're more likely to stick with it. You can do this on deniseaustin.com.

8. Slip on your workout clothes and don't take them off until you sweat. This is one of the biggest things I do to stay motivated (yes, even *I* have trouble at times). The second I wake up, I put on my workout clothes and sneakers because I know that I'd be embarrassed to take them off without squeezing in a workout.

9. TV can be another motivator. I like to watch ESPN (with the sound turned off while listening to music) because all those athletes get me psyched up. But you can also record your favorite shows and work out while watching, or use the commercials to do exercises such as squats, crunches, and push-ups.

10. Make healthy foods look more appetizing and thus more satisfying. Instead of eating yogurt out of the container, put it in a bowl and alternate layers of yogurt and fruit, or make fish and veggies more appealing by adding a garnish of mint or parsley.

11. Keep a food log. Studies show that people who kept food journals lost more weight than those who didn't. Also, knowing that you have to jot down what you put in your mouth can prevent mindless eating and inspire you to choose healthy options.

12. Remind yourself that you'll *always, always* feel better after you exercise than you did before you started (or if you skip it)!

MONDAY'S DAILY DOZEN MEAL PLANS

*There's no time like the present.
We are going to make healthy food choices today!*

Week One Monday Daily Dozen Meal Plan

I hope you love today's Feta & Cranberry Salad for lunch! I do. Dried cranberries add sweetness to this midday meal and are full of antioxidants, compounds that can help stave off many diseases. These little dried berries tossed with protein-rich turkey and feta cheese make a salad a filling meal. And that's key. I know lots of people think surviving on salads is the way to lose weight, but unless a salad is topped with some protein and healthy fat, you'll find yourself ravenous shortly after you eat it. I also know that you're going to enjoy tonight's Maple Glazed Grilled Salmon, a dish my whole family loves because it's sweet and filling at the same time. Of course, I like it because it's rich in omega-3 fatty acids, which reduce inflammation in the body and in turn help protect against so many things—from arthritis to wrinkles.

BREAKFAST
1 egg + 2 egg whites scrambled
   with ¼ cup chopped
   bell pepper (2 protein +
   ¼ veggie)
1 slice whole wheat bread,
   toasted (1 grain)
1 medium orange (1 fruit)

LUNCH
Feta & Cranberry Salad
   (3½ veggie + 1 protein +
   ½ fruit + 2 healthy fat)
1 medium banana (1 fruit)

Feta & Cranberry Salad

3 cups baby spinach
½ cup chopped cucumber
2 ounces roasted turkey breast
2 tablespoons crumbled low-fat feta cheese
2 tablespoons dried cranberries
2 teaspoons extra-virgin olive oil
2 teaspoons balsamic vinegar

In a large bowl, combine the spinach, cucumber, turkey, feta, and cranberries. Drizzle with oil and vinegar.

Maple Glazed Grilled Salmon

2 teaspoons maple syrup
1 tablespoon reduced-sodium soy sauce
Women: 3 ounces grilled salmon
Men: 5 ounces grilled salmon

Preheat the grill. Combine the maple syrup and soy sauce in a small bowl. Place the salmon skin-side down on the grill and brush the sauce combination on top. Grill for approximately 10 minutes per inch of thickness or until cooked all the way through.

AFTERNOON SNACK
2 tablespoons unsalted
    almonds (1 healthy fat)
1 medium apple (1 fruit)

DINNER
Maple Glazed Grilled Salmon
    (*women:* 1 protein; *men:*
    1½ protein)
¾ cup cooked brown rice
    (¾ grain)
¾ cup steamed mixed
    vegetables (¾ veggie)

NUTRITION INFORMATION FOR THE DAY:

WOMEN	MEN
Calories: 1,248 kcal	*Calories:* 1,504 kcal
Total Fat: 35 g	*Total Fat:* 46 g
Saturated Fat: 8 g	*Saturated Fat:* 9 g
Total Carbohydrate: 163 g	*Total Carbohydrate:* 182 g
Protein: 76 g	*Protein:* 96 g
Sodium: 1,708 mg	*Sodium:* 1,759 mg
Fiber: 26 g	*Fiber:* 31 g

DAILY DOZEN TOTALS FOR THE DAY:

WOMEN	MEN
4 protein	4½ protein
4½ veggie	4½ veggie
3½ fruit	3½ fruit
1¾ grain	1¾ grain
3 healthy fat	3 healthy fat

Week Two Monday Daily Dozen Meal Plan

Today's 4 Minute Grains for breakfast is something I came up with years ago. It's one of my favorite morning meals when I need something hearty. I love how it fills me up and contains oats and barley, which have so many cholesterol-lowering benefits. They also help regulate your blood sugar, which keeps you feeling full longer and, over the long term, prevents diabetes. And get ready for a yummy dinner that doesn't feel like a diet: the Awesome Chicken Brick Burger. You'll love it and so will everyone else.

BREAKFAST
4 Minute Grains (1 grain +
    1 fruit + ½ healthy fat)
1 banana (1 fruit)

MORNING SNACK
10 baby carrots (1 veggie)
¼ cup hummus (1 protein +
    ½ healthy fat)
Men add: ¼ cup hummus
    and 2 hard-boiled egg
    whites (1 protein + 1 healthy
    fat)

LUNCH
Turkey & Avocado Wrap
    (1 grain + 1 protein + 1
    veggie + ½ healthy fat)
1 medium apple (1 fruit)
Men add: 1 medium apple
    (1 fruit)

AFTERNOON SNACK
½ cup nonfat Greek yogurt
    (½ protein)

4 Minute Grains

3 tablespoons quick-cooking barley
3 tablespoons Irish oatmeal
⅔ cup water
Ground cinnamon, to taste
¼ cup raisins (or any dried fruit)
1 tablespoon raw walnuts

Combine the barley, oats, and water in a microwave-safe bowl and microwave for 2 minutes. Add the cinnamon and raisins and microwave for 2 more minutes. Top with walnuts and serve.

Turkey & Avocado Wrap

1 whole wheat wrap
3 ounces roasted turkey breast
2 handfuls baby spinach
4 slices cucumber
2 tablespoons diced avocado

Place the wrap on a plate and layer the ingredients inside. Roll up and enjoy!

½ cup mixed berries (½ fruit)

Men add: ½ cup mixed berries (½ fruit)

DINNER

Awesome Chicken Brick Burger (*women:* 1 protein + 1 veggie; *men:* 1 protein + 2 veggies)

Awesome Chicken Brick Burger

4 ounces ground chicken breast
2 tablespoons panko bread crumbs
1 scallion, chopped
½ teaspoon minced garlic
¼ teaspoon Asian hot chili sauce
1 tablespoon bottled teriyaki sauce
1 teaspoon honey
¼ teaspoon canola oil
1 cup arugula
Men add: 1 cup arugula

Except for the oil and arugula, mix all the ingredients in a large bowl. Then form the mixture into a patty. Add the oil to your pan or grill, heat, and place the patty on the hot pan. Place a brick that is clean and wrapped in foil on top of the burger to press. Cook for about 3 to 4 minutes, flip, and continue cooking for about 3 minutes more until cooked through. Serve the burger over arugula.

NUTRITION INFORMATION FOR THE DAY:

WOMEN	MEN
Calories: 1,263 kcal	*Calories:* 1,426 kcal
Total Fat: 21 g	*Total Fat:* 27 g
Saturated Fat: 5 g	*Saturated Fat:* 6 g
Total Carbohydrate: 197 g	*Total Carbohydrate:* 214 g
Protein: 78 g	*Protein:* 87 g
Sodium: 1,187 mg	*Sodium:* 1,424 mg
Fiber: 23 g	*Fiber:* 29 g

DAILY DOZEN TOTALS FOR THE DAY:

WOMEN	MEN
3½ protein	4½ protein
3 veggie	4 veggie
3½ fruit	5 fruit
2 grain	2 grain
1½ healthy fat	2½ healthy fat

Week Three Monday Daily Dozen Meal Plan

Today's breakfast is one of my personal favorite creations, 4 Minute Grains, which we had for breakfast last Monday as well—but this time we'll add a glass of skim milk for extra protein. It's a blend of fiber-rich barley and Irish oats, both of which make this morning meal slimming and filling. Plus, it contains raisins, a good source of iron, and walnuts, a fabulous source of vitamin E, antioxidants, and alpha-linolenic acid. The latter is one of the omega-3 fatty acids that's great for your heart as well as your complexion and your hair. I also love this Quick Salmon Salad for lunch. It's another way to get your fill of those important omega-3 fatty acids. Canned salmon is great, but sometimes in summer I'll use leftover grilled salmon from the night before. And dinner's Beef & Broccoli Stir-Fry gives you the tasty flavor of Chinese takeout without the fat, calories, and MSG.

MAKE EATING OUT DIET-FRIENDLY

Don't be afraid to ask questions when dining out! It's up to you to make healthy choices, not your waiter. Ask what ingredients entrées contain and how foods are prepared. And never be afraid to ask for changes in your order like salad dressing on the side, a dish cooked with less oil, or the chance to substitute something fattening like french fries or a mayo-based salad with steamed veggies, a salad, or fruit. Remember: You are paying for your meal; you should get what you want!

Quick Salmon Salad

½ cup boneless canned salmon
1 teaspoon extra-virgin olive oil
1 tablespoon lemon juice
1 teaspoon minced red onion
1 teaspoon chopped fresh parsley
1 teaspoon capers, rinsed and drained
1 teaspoon red wine vinegar
Salt and pepper, to taste
2 cups mixed greens

In a medium bowl, combine all ingredients except the greens; toss to combine. Serve over mixed greens.

Beef & Broccoli Stir-Fry

1 teaspoon canola oil
1 clove garlic, minced
1 teaspoon freshly grated ginger
4 ounces flank steak, thinly sliced
1 cup chopped broccoli
½ cup sliced red onion
1 tablespoon reduced-sodium soy sauce
1 teaspoon Chinese five-spice powder

Heat the oil in a large wok or skillet over medium-high heat. Add the garlic, ginger, and steak; toss and cook for about 2 minutes. Add the broccoli, onion, soy sauce, and five-spice powder. Continue to stir-fry until the broccoli is bright green and slightly tender.

BREAKFAST

4 Minute Grains (see recipe on page 85) (1 grain + 1 fruit + ½ healthy fat)
1 cup skim milk (1 protein)
Men add: 1 cup grapes (1 fruit)

MORNING SNACK

1 tablespoon natural peanut butter (I like Smucker's Natural Peanut Butter) (½ healthy fat)
6 whole wheat crackers (1 grain)

LUNCH

Quick Salmon Salad (1 protein + 1 healthy fat + 2 veggie)
1 medium banana (1 fruit)

AFTERNOON SNACK

1 medium apple (1 fruit)

DINNER

Beef & Broccoli Stir-Fry (1 protein + 1½ veggie)
½ cup cooked brown rice (½ grain)
Men add: ½ cup cooked brown rice (½ grain)

NUTRITION INFORMATION FOR THE DAY:

WOMEN	MEN
Calories: 1,380 kcal	*Calories:* 1,676 kcal
Total Fat: 41 g	*Total Fat:* 51 g
Saturated Fat: 8 g	*Saturated Fat:* 10 g
Total Carbohydrate: 184 g	*Total Carbohydrate:* 232 g
Protein: 81 g	*Protein:* 88 g
Sodium: 1,514 mg	*Sodium:* 1,535 mg
Fiber: 24 g	*Fiber:* 28 g

DAILY DOZEN TOTALS FOR THE DAY:

WOMEN	MEN
3 protein	3 protein
3½ veggie	3½ veggie
3 fruit	4 fruit
2½ grain	3 grain
2 healthy fat	2 healthy fat

TRUE BEAUTY DOESN'T COME FROM A BOTTLE

What I find beautiful is a person who takes care of herself by eating well and exercising regularly. It's not about crow's-feet or a few extra pounds. You can't bottle and apply the glow of good health or the look of confidence that feeling good about yourself radiates. It comes from within, and you can develop it yourself.

A Dozen Tips from Denise: Twelve Ways to Trim Your Body and Your Food Costs

I often hear people say that eating healthy is too expensive, but I disagree. Sure, some fast food costs less than a dollar. But it's not worth it to eat all that heart-clogging fat and high-calorie food, especially when there are some easy ways to make healthy foods fit your budget and watch your waistline and your wallet. Here, some of my favorite tips:

1. Buy in bulk. I buy whole grains, nuts, dried beans, oats, dried fruits, and organic brown rice in bulk at places like Costco, Sam's Club, and BJ's. Because you're not paying for extra packaging or marketing, your price per pound is a lot cheaper.

2. Don't buy small packages. It may be easier to buy portion-size packages of food, but those little bags are often more expensive. Instead, I suggest buying the large package—say, of crackers or pretzels—and then dividing it into small portions in individual plastic bags when you get home. (They even make hundred-calorie plastic bags, which make it a cinch to eat healthy on a dime!)

3. Shop locally. I go to a store in my area called the Mediterranean Bakery because it's a great bargain. I buy local produce and very reasonably priced olive oil there. I also go to my local farmer's market on Saturday mornings. It's fresh and wholesome, less expensive, and you're supporting local farmers.

4. Buy seasonally. I plan my recipes and weekly menus around what's currently in season. These foods are lower in price and typically have much better flavor, too.

5. Grow your own. Homegrown is always best. I have my own herb garden in my kitchen. I can take snips of what I need, like fresh basil, thyme, parsley, and rosemary, and it costs me just pennies.

6. Cook yourself. Restaurant meals tend to be pricier than what you'd eat at home, plus you don't know exactly what goes into them so it's harder to track fat and calories. I love to cook at home because I can control exactly what ingredients are in my food—such as how much salt or oil is used—as well as portion size. I also know that there are no preservatives, something you can't guarantee at fast-food or other restaurants.

7. Pick inexpensive edibles. Foods that give you more nutritional bang for your buck include potatoes, beans, eggs, milk, and canned tuna and soups. These foods have low price tags but are high in vitamins, minerals, and other healthy compounds. Did you know an Idaho potato only costs about a quarter?

8. Split costs with a friend. Sometimes the food at those warehouse stores *is* less expensive but comes in huge packages that you can't possibly finish. Instead, find a friend to split some of these items with.

9. Make restaurant meals more cost-efficient. Today's restaurant meals are bigger than ever. Instead of eating too much and regretting it later or wasting food, have your waiter put half your entrée in a to-go box before he even brings it to the table. For one price, you get dinner today and another meal for tomorrow!

10. Cook in bulk. Once you're chopping, dicing, and cooking, why not make more than one meal at once and then freeze it or put it in the fridge for another day? This certainly saves time, but it also saves money since those veggies or other perishable items you bought to cook won't go to waste.

11. Brown-bag your lunch. Even if you do have a healthy place to buy food at work, it's always cheaper to bring your own. This way, you're not paying marked-up prices for something like a sandwich or salad that you could easily make yourself at home.

12. Practice good food storage. There's nothing worse than spending good money on healthy foods only to find yourself tossing rotten, unused items like fruits and veggies at the end of the week. Use your refrigerator's crisper drawers for vegetables, and when you freeze foods make sure the containers you use are made for the freezer (this helps ward off freezer burn and loss of flavor).

TWELVE WAYS TO SPICE UP YOUR WATER

Plain H_2O can get boring, but drinking enough water is critical when you're trying to lose weight. To make sure you drink a lot throughout the day, keep a full bottle with you at all times and sip often. You can also make it a bit more exciting and appetizing by adding one of the following to a big jug of water you keep in the fridge to sip throughout the day. I feel like I'm at a spa when I do this, and it makes it a lot easier to drink the required eight glasses of water a day.

1. Slices of cucumber (I love the seedless ones!).

2. Orange wedges.

3. Shredded ginger.

4. Mint leaves.

5. Chopped strawberries.

6. Two splashes of grapefruit juice.

7. Lemon slices.

8. A peppermint tea bag.

9. Green tea drops (available at most health food stores).

10. A teaspoon of cranberry juice.

11. Celery sticks.

12. Ice cubes made from orange juice.

My Daily Dozen Monday Checklist

	WEEK ONE	WEEK TWO	WEEK THREE
I ate my Daily Dozen Foods			
VEGGIE			
VEGGIE			
VEGGIE			
FRUIT			
FRUIT			
FRUIT			
PROTEIN			
PROTEIN			
PROTEIN			
HEALTHY GRAIN			
HEALTHY GRAIN			
HEALTHY FAT			
EIGHT 8-OUNCE GLASSES OF WATER			
I did my Daily Dozen exercises			
I did some of my weekly twelve miles of cardio (write how many miles)			
I did some fidget-cisers today (write how many)			

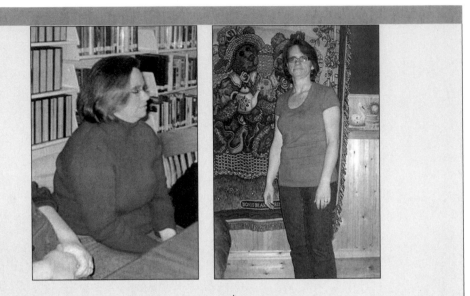

Rhonda Duell,

37, assistant librarian, Shinglehouse, Pennsylvania

POUNDS LOST: 45

At 189 pounds, I was self-conscious, depressed, and uncomfortable in my body. So on my thirty-sixth birthday, I decided it was time for a change. I set a goal to enter my forties in better shape than I was in my thirties. I felt excited that I was going to take charge of my life, even if I was overwhelmed by the amount of weight I had to lose. One thing I knew for sure: This time I didn't want to 'diet' in order to lose the weight. I had tried diets in my early thirties. They were great as long as I stuck to them, but when I'd lost what I wanted to lose and went off the diet, all the weight came back—and then some! This time I needed a lifestyle change, not a diet. That's what I found with Denise's plan.

"I used to drink soda all day long, but gave it up and now I drink mostly water, at least a hundred ounces a day. I also try to choose fruits and vegetable more often, instead of sweets. I exercise at least half an hour a day, six days a week, and make sure I change my exercise routine monthly. I have a lot of Denise's exercise workouts on tape and DVD, and that gives me variety so I don't get bored. So far, I have lost forty-five pounds! And my cholesterol has also come down from 268 to 167 so I no longer have to take the high blood pressure medicine I was on for thirteen years! I still have more weight to lose, but I know I'll be able to do it. Thanks to Denise, I'm more confident and less self-conscious. I have so much more energy and I'm able to keep up with my five kids and a full-time job!"

Tuesday

Welcome to Tuesday! Another day to get fit, feel terrific, and move closer to the shape and fitness level that you want to—and *can*—achieve. I've always liked the saying "You can do anything that you set your mind to," and it's certainly true when it comes to losing weight and shaping up. I'm a big believer in facing each day with a positive attitude, focusing on what you can do and what you can control, and moving forward from there. Remember that you deserve to be fit and feel great (and look good in your jeans, too!). Beyond that, you're going to be healthier, and that's worth every second that you exercise or seek out foods that are good for you. Keep focused on your goals, stay positive, and by this time next week you'll start to notice big changes—be it pounds lost, looser-fitting clothes, increased energy, or all of the above.

Tuesday's Daily Dozen workout focuses on your lower body and abs. These two areas tend to be trouble spots for a lot of people, so the twelve easy exercises are some of the most effective and efficient for targeting the hips, thighs, and buttocks. They'll trim those saddlebags, lift your rear, tighten up those jiggling thighs, and whittle your middle. These are the exercises that I do to keep my own

TAKE IT SLOW

Resist the urge to cheat and use momentum to keep going with your exercises. I know it's tempting to rush through your workout, especially if you find part of your routine particularly challenging. But trust me, you'll get the most bang for your body if you keep a slow-and-steady pace—consistency pays off. You're doing great!

NOBODY'S PERFECT

Like me, I'm sure you always try your hardest to stay on top of things, but sometimes you get derailed. An unexpected phone call leaves you running fifteen minutes late. One of your children stays home from school with a cold, and you need to stay home, too. Or you have lunch with a friend and overeat that chocolate mousse. Then what happens? You get mad at yourself. You aim for perfection and then get upset when you miss the mark. And that's negativity you just don't need! We all make mistakes (it's human!), but you can't let those slipups get the best of you. Don't get discouraged if you eat junk or miss a workout—and certainly don't throw in the towel! Plan to do better tomorrow: Do an extra twelve-minute Daily Dozen workout or walk a little bit farther. You can do it!

lower body in shape, so I know that they work. Today's Daily Dozen includes lunges and squats, two moves that research has shown are the best ones to tone your rear—and they're moves you can do almost anywhere. In fact, I often do them while brushing my teeth or standing at the stove (see Twelve Favorite Fidget-cisers on page 16). Also, like the majority of the exercises in the Daily Dozen, many of Tuesday's moves do more than tone and firm your body. For example, the seated thigh toner strengthens the muscles in front of your thighs above the kneecap (called the quadriceps), which helps ward off very common—but painful—knee injuries. And the plank is a major multitasker because it simultaneously works your legs, butt, abs, and arms. And here's more inspiring news for you: Tuesday's Daily Dozen lower-body exercises can even help reduce the appearance of cellulite. (I thought that would get your attention.) But enough talking, let's get going. Just grab your two sets of dumbbells and exercise mat and get ready to slim down below the waist.

Knowledge is power! The more you learn about your body, the stronger you'll be!

Reshape and transform your bottom half to make it your better half! Get firm and lose the flab. You'll lose inches because fat takes up five times more space than muscle.

1. Warm Up

▶ SQUAT WITH OUTER THIGH: Stand with your feet shoulder-width apart, your hands on your thighs, and squat down. As you stand up, alternate swinging your legs straight out to the side. Time: 30 seconds.

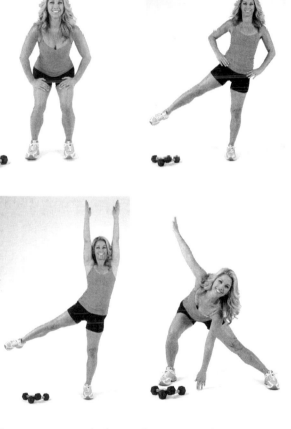

▶ CHALLENGE: Repeat the squat while lifting your arms straight up and down over your head.

▶ INNER-THIGH STRETCH: Stand with your legs three to four feet apart and your toes facing forward. Lunge to the right, keeping your weight on your right leg. Place your left hand on the ground and twist your upper body, extending the right arm toward the ceiling. Switch sides and repeat. Time: 30 seconds.

2. Squats

Remember that your rear end is the last thing to leave the room,
so make a good lasting impression.

▶ DOUBLE-LEG SQUAT: Holding a weight in each hand, stand with your feet a little wider than your hips and your arms by the sides of your body, elbows slightly bent.

▶ Squat down, sitting way back and keeping your body weight through your heels. Squeeze your buttocks as you straighten your legs to the start position, then repeat. Time: 1 minute.

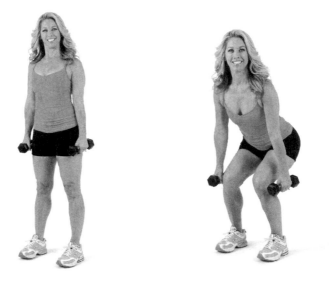

▶ CHALLENGE: Single-leg squat: When you squat, lift the heel of the left foot off the ground, balancing only on the left toe. Sit all your weight into your right leg, keeping your back strong and abs pulled in. Switch legs and repeat.

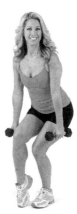

3. Lunge Series
Stubborn cellulite be gone!

▶ Hold a dumbbell in each hand with your arms extended straight down by your sides, back straight, and abs pulled in.

▶ Step your left leg behind you about three feet. Then bend your right knee so it's at a ninety-degree angle, with the left knee pointing down toward the floor.

▶ Push off your back leg, using the right thigh and butt cheek to lift it off the floor, bringing the left knee in front of you to hip height. Make sure to pull your abs in every time you lift your knee. Switch legs and repeat. Time: 1 minute.

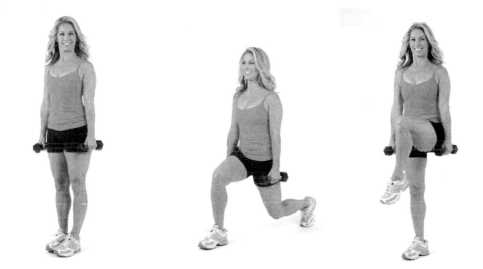

▶ CHALLENGE: Add a curtsy when you bring the leg back behind you

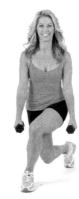

4. Deadlift

Kiss that flabby butt good-bye! And firm up the backs of your thighs.
No more "cottage cheese" look!

▶ Hold a dumbbell in each hand with your arms down in front of your body. Stand nice and tall with your feet hip-width apart, knees slightly bent.

▶ Keeping your abs strong and back straight the whole time, slowly bend forward at your hips to lower the weights toward the floor with your hands directly under your shoulders. Then return to standing as you squeeze your buttocks and thighs (it's this squeeze that really helps lift and shape this area). Time: 1 minute.

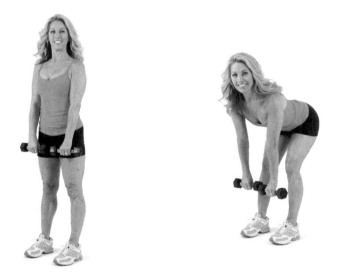

▶ CHALLENGE: As you bring your body weight down in front of you and reach toward the floor, extend one leg straight off the ground behind you. Alternate which leg you lift each time.

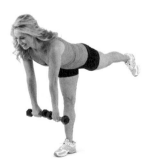

5. Side Lunge

You'll love this great outer-thigh slimmer.

▶ Stand with your feet shoulder-width apart and hold a dumbbell in each hand with your arms extended straight down in front of your body.

▶ Step out to the right side about three to four feet and lunge down with the right leg. Return to standing and repeat on the left side. Continue alternating side lunges. Time: 1 minute.

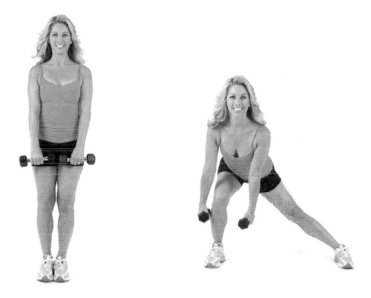

▶ CHALLENGE: As you stand up out of each side lunge, bend the right knee and lift the right leg up to hip height before doing the next lunge.

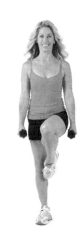

6. Seated Thigh Toner
Zap flab above the knee fast.

▸ Sit with your back straight and tall with your left leg extended straight. Bend your right leg and place your right foot flat on the floor. Rest your hands on your left knee to help you keep good posture.

▸ With your left foot flexed, lift and lower your leg. Do all reps on one leg, then switch legs and repeat. Time: 30 seconds per leg.

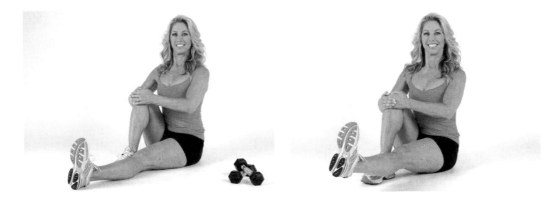

▸ CHALLENGE: Turn your foot slightly out to the side to about two o'clock for the right foot and ten o'clock for the left.

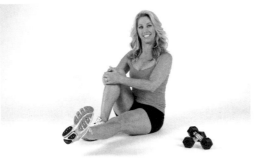

7. Plank with Back of Thigh Firmer

Need a move to sculpt you head-to-toe? This is it!

▶ Position your body in a plank, balancing on your toes and hands. If this is too challenging, position yourself on your knees and forearms.

▶ While holding your tummy up and in, bend your left leg, bringing your flexed foot toward your rear in a hamstring curl. Complete all the reps on one leg and then switch legs and repeat. Time: 30 seconds per leg.

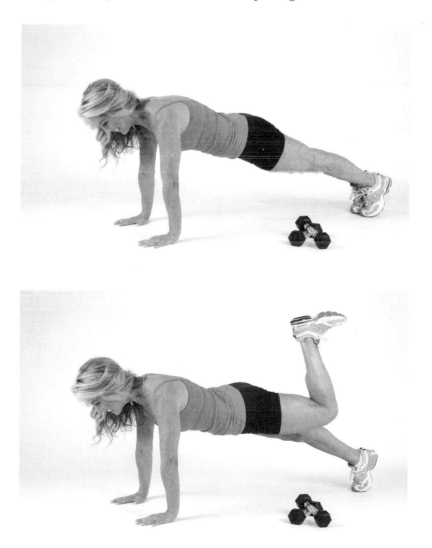

8. Leg Circles with Core

This zeros in on your hips, outer thighs, and core,
creating lean legs and a taut tummy!

▸ Kneeling on the ground, lean over to your left and place your left hand on the floor. Place your right hand on your hip, lift your right leg off the floor, and straighten it at hip height. Make small circles with your leg. Complete all reps on one side, then switch legs and repeat. Time: 30 seconds per leg.

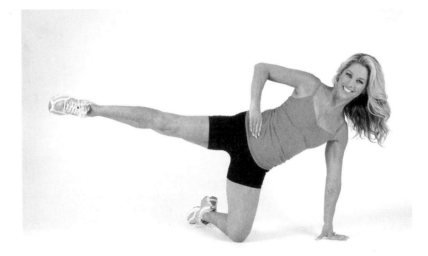

▸ CHALLENGE: Take the hand off your hip and extend it straight toward the ceiling. Look toward your hand.

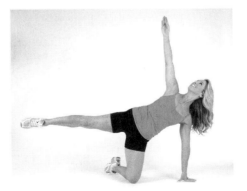

9. Butt Blaster

Sculpt and carve a rounded, beautiful rear. Make your backside your best side.

▸ Position your body so that you're on the floor on your hands and knees. Place one dumbbell behind your bent left knee.

▸ Flex your foot and lift your left leg up toward the ceiling, then down toward the floor. Keep your back strong and pull your abs up and in as you lift your leg. Complete all reps on your left leg, then switch legs and repeat. Time: 30 seconds per leg.

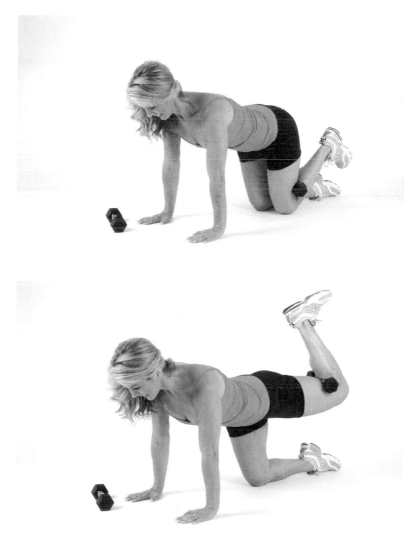

10. Bicycle

The American Council on Exercise rated this as the best ab move you can do.
It targets all the ab muscles.

▶ Lie on your back with your legs bent and in the air so that you form a ninety-degree angle between your torso and thighs. Place your hands behind your head with your elbows open out to the sides, tighten your abs, and lift your upper torso so that your shoulder blades hover just off the floor. Keeping your neck and shoulders relaxed, twist your upper body to the left side, bringing your left knee toward your right elbow while extending your right leg a few inches off the floor. Switch sides, bringing your left elbow toward your right knee and extending your left leg a few inches off the floor. Time: 1 minute.

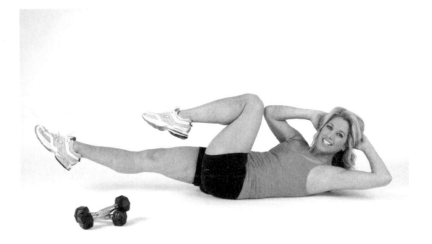

11. Inner-Thigh Toner

No more inner-high jiggle. Did you know the inner thighs are among the most underused muscles in the body? This move targets and tones them.

▶ Lie on your back with your legs bent and feet flat on the floor. Place a hand towel between your knees and squeeze. Rest your arms by the sides of your body with your palms on the floor.

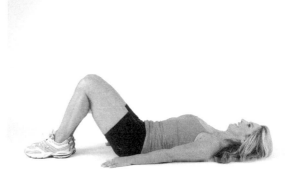

▶ Squeeze your legs together and lift your hips up off the floor. Lift and lower your hips. Time: 30 seconds.

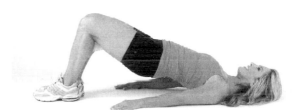

▶ Extend your right leg straight at the same height as your thighs. Hold and squeeze your inner thighs together. Time: 15 seconds. Switch legs and repeat.

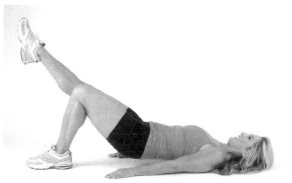

12. Cool-Down Stretches

▸ HIP/BUTT: Sit on the floor with your legs extended straight in front of you. Place your hands behind you with the palms down and fingers facing your body. Lift your hips and butt up off the floor and straighten your arms. Elongate the legs and stretch out the chest as you hold.

▸ HIP/BUTT: Lie on your back with your legs bent, feet flat on the floor. Lift your legs off the floor and place your right ankle across your left knee. Use the left leg to press the right leg toward your body. Switch legs and repeat.

▸ HAMSTRING STRETCH: Lie on your back with your legs bent, feet flat on the floor. Lift your right leg off the floor and place your hands behind your knee as you straighten the leg and pull it toward your chest. Switch legs and repeat.

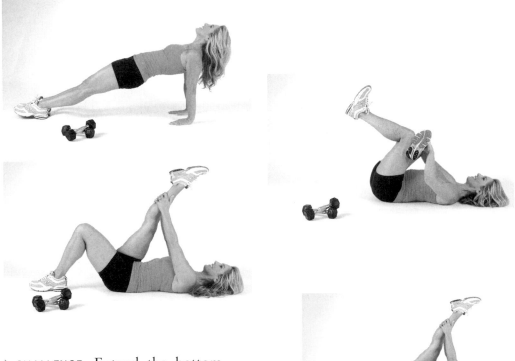

▸ CHALLENGE: Extend the bottom leg straight on the floor while doing the hamstring stretch.

A Dozen Tips from Denise: Easy Ways to Boost Your Energy

The world we live in is go-go-go all the time. However, sometimes all that going leaves us feeling wiped out and in need of a major energy boost. I'm happy to say there are many healthy ways to get that lift, and most of them take just a few minutes out of your day. Here, some of my favorite ways to feel revived and refreshed.

1. Research shows that the scents of citrus and peppermint can make you feel more energized and alert. Light up a lemon- or mint-fragranced candle, rub on orange or peppermint lotion, or sip some citrus or peppermint tea.

2. Breathe. Taking some long deep breaths is a simple way to give yourself an energy boost no matter where you are. Try inhaling for the count of three and exhaling for the count of three. Repeat several times.

3. Good posture also has an impact on your energy level, because how you sit affects how much oxygen can flow through your body. For example, if you sit at a desk all day, often by 3 PM your shoulders are hunched forward and your back is rounded. With that kind of slouched posture, your breathing tends to be shallow—and that means less oxygen is flowing through your body and to your brain. No wonder you're tired! On the other hand, having good posture helps increase your lung capacity, which leaves you feeling more alert. So sit up tall, stretch your arms out to the sides, and look up to the ceiling as you lean slightly back, open your chest, and do the deep breathing recommended above.

4. One of the first things I do when my energy is fading is to drink water. Every cell in our bodies needs water to function at its best, so it makes sense that being dehydrated may slow you down. Grab a bottle of water when you need a lift. (For ideas on how to spice up your H_2O and make it more appealing, see page 92.)

5. One of the most important ways to keep your energy up throughout the day is to keep your blood sugar level stable. That's why I never go longer than three to four hours without eating (and why starvation diets leave you feeling exhausted). Even if it's just something small—a handful of almonds, some yogurt, or an apple—it will keep your metabolism going strong and give you the energy you need to get through your busy day.

6. Always eat breakfast. This is along the lines of not going too long without eating. When you wake up in the morning, it's likely been at least eight hours since you've eaten—in fact, the word *breakfast* really means to "break the fast"—so your body needs some fuel to give it a kick start. Skip breakfast and you'll start your day behind the eight ball and be starving come noon.

7. Skip the sugar. When you're exhausted, it's easy to reach for a sugary snack like cookies or candy thinking it will give you the boost you need. At first it does increase your blood sugar level, so you do feel a little better. The problem is that soon enough, your blood sugar level falls drastically and you're back to feeling wiped out again. Instead, eat plenty of protein *and* carbs, because this combination keeps your energy up and leaves you feeling full longer.

8. Get enough vitamin B_6. This nutrient is necessary for a variety of functions in the body such as protein metabolism and proper functioning of your nervous and immune systems. It also helps keep your blood sugar levels stable, which, as I mentioned earlier, is critical if you want to feel alert and wide-eyed. Look for foods that contain B_6, including fortified cereals and oatmeal, baked potatoes (make sure to eat the skin), bananas, garbanzo beans, and chicken.

9. This may sound obvious, but getting enough rest is key. I'm a big believer in getting seven to eight hours of sleep a night—if you're not rested, you'll feel worn out before your day even starts. (See page 141 for tips on improving your sleep.)

10. Eating spinach is another one of my personal energy-boosting tricks. (Yes, Popeye was on to something when he professed his love for this green, leafy vegetable!) It's a rich source of some amazing nutrients like iron (something most women don't get enough of), folic acid, vitamins A, C, E, and K, magnesium, calcium, and an array of antioxidants. I love it in a salad, lightly steamed, or added to a wrap or sandwich.

11. Rub your ears. I learned this trick about twenty years ago when I was on a plane flying cross-country. A very interesting doctor I was sitting next to told me that a great way to feel more alert and calm was to use two fingers to gently press down all along the perimeter of your ear. She also suggested rubbing the back of the hard bony part of the ear. I know it sounds a little crazy, but I've been doing it for two decades now so I know it works!

12. Laugh often. You may be, well, laughing at this one, but it's true. Cracking up helps get oxygen flowing through your body and raises your heart rate, all of which can perk you up. So call your funniest friend or watch a silly clip on YouTube and you'll be energized in no time.

Be kind to your body, and it will be kind back!

Week One Tuesday Daily Dozen Meal Plan

Breakfast today feels like an indulgent dessert—without the fat and calories. The fruits it contains—mangoes and strawberries—are bursting with vitamins that boost your immune system and also enhance collagen production so your skin looks and feels younger. I know eating chicken when you're trying to lose weight can get boring, but that's not the case with the cilantro and lime chicken dish that you'll have for dinner. It's delicious and loaded with protein to help repair and strengthen your muscles after the hard work you did for today's Daily Dozen.

BREAKFAST

Yogurt Parfait (1 protein +
  1 fruit + 1 healthy fat)
1 slice sprouted grain bread
  (Food for Life brand),
  toasted, with butter spray
  (1 grain)
Men add: 1 slice sprouted grain
  bread (1 grain)

Yogurt Parfait

1 cup nonfat vanilla yogurt
½ cup sliced strawberries
½ cup sliced mango (fresh or frozen)
2 tablespoons sliced almonds
Lime juice, to taste
Zest of lime

In a glass bowl or tall glass, alternate layers of yogurt with layers of fruit. Top with almonds, a squeeze or two of lime, and garnish with lime zest.

THINK POSITIVE!

Whenever your willpower starts to wane, try shifting your focus from your negative thoughts to thoughts of your loved ones. Make it your goal to set an example for your family and be a role model for your kids or your friends! Think of how much they'll all benefit from learning and following all the healthy habits you've picked up.

Tuna Salad Wrap

3 ounces canned tuna (packed in water, drained)

1 teaspoon light mayonnaise

1 teaspoon Dijon mustard

½ cup chopped celery

1 whole-grain wrap

1 handful mixed greens

In a small bowl, combine the tuna, mayo, mustard, and celery; mix to combine. Place the tuna mixture on top of the whole-grain wrap and top with greens.

Chicken with Cilantro & Lime

1 tablespoon olive or canola oil

1 tablespoon honey

Juice of 1 lime

¼ cup chopped cilantro

4 ounces chicken breast

In a small bowl, whisk together the oil, honey, lime juice, and cilantro. Pour this mixture over the chicken breast and marinate in the refrigerator for 20 minutes. Grill or roast the chicken for 6 to 8 minutes per side or until cooked through.

LUNCH

Tuna Salad Wrap (1 protein + 1½ veggie + 1 grain)

1 medium apple (1 fruit)

Men add: 1 medium apple (1 fruit)

AFTERNOON SNACK

1 cup cantaloupe chunks (1 fruit)

Men add: ½ cup nonfat cottage cheese (1 protein) and 2 tablespoons ground flaxseed (1 healthy fat)

DINNER

Chicken with Cilantro & Lime (1 protein)

1 cup steamed spinach (1 veggie)

Men add: ½ cup steamed spinach (½ veggie)

1 small ear of corn (1 veggie)

NUTRITION INFORMATION FOR THE DAY:

WOMEN	MEN
Calories: 1,144 kcal	*Calories:* 1,462 kcal
Total Fat: 28 g	*Total Fat:* 37 g
Saturated Fat: 4 g	*Saturated Fat:* 4 g
Total Carbohydrate: 150 g	*Total Carbohydrate:* 202 g
Protein: 74 g	*Protein:* 101 g
Sodium: 1,145 mg	*Sodium:* 1,790 mg
Fiber: 23 g	*Fiber:* 42 g

DAILY DOZEN TOTALS FOR THE DAY:

WOMEN	MEN
3 protein	4 protein
3½ veggie	4 veggie
3 fruit	4 fruit
2 grain	3 grain
1 healthy fat	2 healthy fat

Week Two Tuesday Daily Dozen Meal Plan

I'm a huge fan of lentils, which is why I've included them for lunch today. They're rich in protein so they give you energy, keep you satisfied, and repair muscles—all

SIT DOWN FOR BREAKFAST

Some people think that skipping breakfast will help them lose weight, but the opposite is true! People who skip breakfast are more likely to gain weight, according to research. When you start the day with a solid breakfast, you'll be less hungry when lunchtime rolls around, so you'll eat fewer calories—which helps keep your weight under control. Breakfast is also an ideal time to get certain nutrients that may be harder to include later in the day, like all that calcium in your glass of milk. Plus, these days, kids are skipping breakfast more and more; if you eat breakfast regularly, you'll set a great example for your children!

while being low in fat and calories. Tonight's dinner—Fish Tacos—is one of my favorites and something I can whip up and know my family will be excited about. This recipe uses mahi mahi, but I also make them with other types of fish depending on what looks best that day. And today you've also got dessert—a yummy baked apple dish. Believe it or not, it's true what they say about an apple a day keeping the doctor away. New research shows that regularly eating apples may reduce allergy symptoms, while other studies reveal that the pectin they contain can help keep you feeling full.

Egg Sandwich

2 egg whites
1 whole-grain English muffin
2 slices tomato

Scramble the eggs in a nonstick pan. Open the English muffin and toast it. Place one slice of tomato on each English muffin half and top with some of the scrambled eggs.

BREAKFAST
Egg Sandwich (1 protein + ½ veggie + 1 grain)
4 fluid ounces orange juice (1 fruit)
Men add: 4 fluid ounces orange juice (1 fruit)

MORNING SNACK
1 cup chopped melon (1 fruit)

Men add: ½ cup red grapes, ¼ cup blueberries, ¼ cup blackberries (1 fruit)
½ cup nonfat cottage cheese (1 protein)

LUNCH
1½ cups low-sodium lentil soup (1½ protein + 1½ veggie)
2 cups mixed greens (2 veggie)
2 tablespoons vinaigrette salad dressing (no more than 100 calories per
  2-tablespoon serving) (1 healthy fat)
½ cup raspberries (½ fruit)
Men add: 1 slice sprouted grain bread, toasted (butter spray optional) (1 grain)

AFTERNOON SNACK
1 tablespoon natural peanut butter (1 healthy fat)
1 large stalk celery (½ veggie)

DINNER
Fish Tacos (2 protein + 1 veggie + 2 grains)
1 medium apple (1 fruit)

Fish Tacos

4 ounces mahi mahi
1 tablespoon olive oil, divided
Salt and pepper, to taste
1 clove garlic, minced
½ cup canned black beans, rinsed and drained
2 small corn tortillas (5–6 inches in diameter), warmed
1 cup shredded green cabbage
¼ cup salsa

Preheat a grill pan or the broiler. Brush the fish with half the olive oil and season with salt and pepper. Cook the fish for 3 to 4 minutes per side, until it's cooked through; set aside. Heat the remaining oil in a small skillet; add the garlic and black beans and sauté until warmed. Add the cooked fish to the black beans and use a spoon to break up into bite-size pieces. Scoop the mahi mahi and black bean mixture into corn tortillas, topping with shredded cabbage and salsa.

NUTRITION INFORMATION FOR THE DAY:

WOMEN
Calories: 1,300 kcal
Total Fat: 37 g
Saturated Fat: 5 g
Total Carbohydrate: 171 g
Protein: 87 g
Sodium: 1,990 mg
Fiber: 34 g

MEN
Calories: 1,553 kcal
Total Fat: 39 g
Saturated Fat: 5 g
Total Carbohydrate: 210 g
Protein: 94 g
Sodium: 2,090 mg
Fiber: 42 g

DAILY DOZEN TOTALS FOR THE DAY:

WOMEN
5½ protein
5½ veggie
3½ fruit
3 grain
2 healthy fat

MEN
5½ protein
5½ veggie
5½ fruit
4 grain
2 healthy fat

Week Three Tuesday Daily Dozen Meal Plan

Commitment is the willingness to be uncomfortable. It is the willingness to stay on track even if something is too hard or takes too long.

An easy time to get your Daily Dozen requirement of fruits and veggies is at breakfast—especially because you can toss veggies into scrambled eggs or omelets. Today I've included bell peppers, which add many nutrients like vitamins A and C as well as a nice satisfying crunch and come in so many different tasty hues. Red grapes, which you'll also have this morning, are wonderful because they're high in antioxidants, particularly resveratrol, which animal studies suggest is an anti-aging compound, and heart-healthy polyphenols. (These compounds are partly why red wine is touted for its health benefits.) And your morning snack—a fresh kiwi and mango combo—has a high concentration of

REACH OUT AND TOUCH SOMEONE!

Have you been meaning to schedule a movie night with the girls, call up your college roommate, or take your favorite aunt out, but haven't made the time? Well, consider this: Research has shown that women who maintain close ties with other women enjoy such health benefits as lower blood pressure, increased immunity, and even longer life expectancy. Get in the habit of catching up with the women in your life a couple times a week. Even a simple phone call will do the trick. After all, haven't you ever had a blah day, only to get a call from a girlfriend or your sister that cheered you up? Be that person to at least one of your close girlfriends or someone in your family today—both of you will reap the benefits!

vitamin C to bolster your immune system, as well as compounds called carotenoids that are thought to decrease disease—and possibly help keep diabetes at bay. If that weren't enough, the salad for lunch is a powerhouse, too. It's my sister Kristine's recipe. Broccoli is part of the brassica family of vegetables, along with cabbage, kale, and brussels sprouts, all of which provide phytochemicals, vitamins, minerals, and fiber. Recent research suggests that eating more brassica vegetables may reduce your risk of several types of cancer. Lastly, tonight's dinner is a simple meal that contains Swiss chard, which is high in vitamins K, A, and C; chicken, which is a great source of lean protein; and whole wheat pasta, which tastes great and gives you tummy-filling fiber.

BREAKFAST

1 egg + 2 egg whites scrambled with ¼ cup chopped bell pepper (any color is great) (2 protein + ¼ veggie)

1 slice whole wheat bread, toasted (1 grain)

Men add: 1 slice whole wheat bread (1 grain)

½ cup red grapes (½ fruit)

MORNING SNACK

1 cup nonfat vanilla yogurt (1 protein)

½ cup chopped kiwi and mango (½ fruit)

Broccoli Slaw Salad

1 cup packaged broccoli slaw
2 tablespoons slivered almonds
½ cup orange segments (I like the Mandarin
   oranges in a jar)
2 tablespoons raisins
¼ cup crispy chow mein noodles or wonton
   strips
1 tablespoon light ranch salad dressing

Place all the ingredients in a bowl and toss
until well mixed.

LUNCH
Broccoli Slaw Salad (1 veggie
   + 1 fruit + 1 healthy fat)
Men add: 1 whole wheat pita
   (1 grain)

AFTERNOON SNACK
1 medium pear (1 fruit)
1 part-skim mozzarella string
   cheese (1 protein)

DINNER
Grilled Chicken with Whole
   Wheat Pasta (2 veggie +
   1 grain + 1 protein)

Grilled Chicken with Whole Wheat Pasta

1 cup frozen mixed vegetables
1 cup cooked whole wheat pasta
1 cup chopped Swiss chard
Salt and black pepper, to taste
Red pepper flakes, to taste
Dried oregano, to taste
Dried basil, to taste
3 ounces grilled chicken breast

Cook the frozen vegetables according to package instructions and set aside. Cook
the pasta according to the directions on the box. Just before the pasta is done,
add the Swiss chard and mixed vegetables to the water and cook for 20 seconds.
When the pasta is done cooking, drain, reserving ¼ cup of the cooking liquid. Transfer the reserved liquid to a bowl and season with salt, pepper, red pepper flakes, oregano, and basil. Mix with the pasta-veggie blend, add the grilled chicken, and serve.

NUTRITION INFORMATION FOR THE DAY:

WOMEN

Calories: 1,420 kcal

Total Fat: 29 g

Saturated Fat: 8 g

Total Carbohydrate: 211 g

Protein: 92 g

Sodium: 1,119 mg

Fiber: 31 g

MEN

Calories: 1,701 kcal

Total Fat: 32 g

Saturated Fat: 9 g

Total Carbohydrate: 266 g

Protein: 102 g

Sodium: 1,609 mg

Fiber: 38 g

DAILY DOZEN TOTALS FOR THE DAY:

WOMEN

5 protein

3¼ veggie

3 fruit

2 grain

1 healthy fat

MEN

5 protein

3¼ veggie

3 fruit

4 grain

1 healthy fat

KEEP FITNESS FRESH

If you find yourself feeling a little ho-hum about your workouts, try injecting a little freshness into your routine. You can try new fitness toys like exercise balls or resistance bands, or download a few new songs or buy a new CD. If you really want to treat yourself, splurge on a new MP3 player or iPod since music is a great get-fit motivator. Of course there are no-cost ways to shake things up, too: Change where you work out (if you're in the gym, head outdoors; if you work out outdoors, try my DVDs at home), the time of day you work out, or whom you exercise with. You'll be amazed how a few small changes can get you psyched up about breaking a sweat.

A Dozen Tips from Denise: Healthy Lunch Options

When you're on the go during the day, you can still have a healthy lunch! Here are some quick (and tasty!) options for brown-bag and store-bought lunches. And if you don't have time to make a complete lunch at home, bring some of the ingredients with you and purchase the rest during the day. It's simple! Keep this lunch list nearby so you always have some healthful, on-the-fly ideas!

Bring these from home:

1. Leftover soup, hummus, and cut-up veggies.

2. Cooked chicken breast on whole-grain bread and low-fat cottage cheese.

3. Hard-boiled eggs and berries or other fruit.

4. Natural peanut butter and jelly on whole-grain bread, cheese slices, and grapes.

5. Lean turkey wrap, a few tortilla chips, and salsa.

6. Low-fat yogurt, a cup of sliced fruit, and ¼ cup whole-grain cereal.

Buy these on the go:

1. Side salad with red kidney beans, balsamic dressing, and soy chips.

2. Miso or vegetable soup and a whole fruit.

3. Grilled chicken salad and a hundred-calorie snack pack.

4. Small tuna salad on greens or spinach, and fruit-flavored yogurt.

5. Sashimi or sushi and fruit salad.

6. Steamed vegetables and brown rice.

TWELVE KEY KITCHEN ESSENTIALS

It's amazing how just a few kitchen items can make eating well and losing weight a lot easier. You probably already have many of the tools listed below, but if you don't they're all inexpensive and well worth adding to your healthy-eating arsenal.

1. Good cutting knives. You don't need pricey knives or a lot of them, but you do need a few that work well. They make food prep such as chopping and slicing fruits, vegetables, and lean protein a lot faster and more enjoyable.

2. Small plastic bags and/or containers. These help you divide food into appropriate portions, something that's especially helpful when you're trying to watch your weight. On Sunday, I often cook up batches of food like hard-boiled eggs and store them in individual bags that I can grab when I'm running out. When I come home from the store with boxes of cereal or snack foods, I divide them up into individual portions. Studies show that we tend to eat more out of big boxes and bags of food. Little bags and containers also make it easy to take healthy snacks and meals on the go, and making your own is more economical than buying pre-packaged snack packs.

3. Measuring spoons and cups. Eventually, you'll be able to eyeball what a tablespoon or half a cup of food looks like, but in the beginning measuring it out can really help you keep calories in check. You'll be surprised to see not only what correct portions are but also how satisfying they can be. With foods I eat regularly, like cereal, I keep a measuring cup in the box so that it's easy to scoop out an accurate portion.

4. Food scale. Not everyone needs one, but if you have trouble figuring out what three ounces of chicken or fish is, it can be really helpful. The good news is that today you can buy a good scale for less than twenty dollars. All you need it for is to weigh your food, so skip the high-priced scales with lots of bells and whistles. That said, if you're someone who likes gadgets, a high-tech version may motivate you to use it more often—and that's good for your waistline.

5. Salad plates, or plates that are seven inches or smaller. It's amazing how the size of the dinner plate has grown over the last twenty to thirty years. The problem with that is we tend to eat more off a larger plate or feel deprived when we see a normal portion of food on a big plate. (Something about all that empty space makes us feel like we're not eating enough.) Trick your eyes and your stomach and teach yourself about appropriate portion sizes by serving meals on smaller plates and bowls.

6. A water pitcher. Having one makes it more likely that you'll actually drink the recommended eight glasses of water than if you have to keep filling your glass from the sink. Also, with a pitcher you can add ingredients like those on page 92 to make yourself a more enticing spa-like drink.

7. A pretty fruit bowl. It doesn't have to be expensive or fancy, just one that you're happy to see on the counter every day. If you fill it with fruit and keep it out, you'll remember to grab a piece of fruit when your tummy starts growling rather than start digging in the pantry.

8. Cheese grater or microplane. I love cheese as much as the next girl, but I also know that too much won't help tip the scale in your favor. When cheese is finely shredded, though, you can sprinkle it on foods like pasta and salads and enjoy its rich flavor without using too much. This works best with cheeses that have a strong flavor like Parmesan and cheddar.

9. Colander. Washing fruits and vegetables before you eat them is important because they may contain pesticides. And even those grown without these chemicals need a scrub-down since they're probably handled a lot from the time they're picked at the farm until they reach your kitchen.

10. Steamer basket. These little metal baskets go inside your pots so that it's easy to steam up vegetables. They cost less than ten dollars at mass merchandisers, department stores, or home stores, yet they cook veggies in a way that makes them tasty and helps them retain their important nutrients.

11. Nonstick pan. Though many oils contain important healthy fats (one of the twelve foods you should eat daily), too much oil can add too many extra calories. With a nonstick pan, you can whip up dishes that are delicious but don't require extra oil or butter.

12. Blender. Sometimes there's nothing more satisfying than a smoothie, and the recipes for these are endless. Blenders are also good for making soups and salad dressings. Though some are pricey, you can definitely find an inexpensive one that will do the trick.

My Daily Dozen Tuesday Checklist

	WEEK ONE	WEEK TWO	WEEK THREE
I ate my Daily Dozen Foods			
VEGGIE			
VEGGIE			
VEGGIE			
FRUIT			
FRUIT			
FRUIT			
PROTEIN			
PROTEIN			
PROTEIN			
HEALTHY GRAIN			
HEALTHY GRAIN			
HEALTHY FAT			
EIGHT 8-OUNCE GLASSES OF WATER			
I did my Daily Dozen exercises			
I did some of my weekly twelve miles of cardio (write how many miles)			
I did some fidget-cisers today (write how many)			

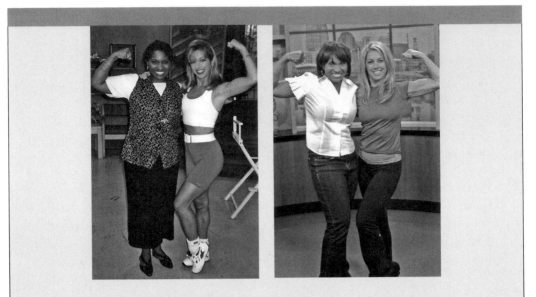

Tuwanda Coleman,
50, television producer, Nashville, Tennessee
POUNDS LOST: 30

I'm a southern Kentucky girl who grew up eating everything prepared with lard and bacon grease. Our breakfasts were as big as dinners, and we never finished a meal without a decadent dessert. By the time I was fourteen, I was forty to fifty pounds overweight. I lost about thirty pounds when I went off to college because I was no longer around my mother's delicious, fattening foods and had to walk two miles up and down a hill to class about three times a day. But once I started working, I slowly started to gain weight, eventually going up to my highest weight of 180 pounds.

"Around this time, I met Denise because I booked her on a talk show I produce in Nashville. I'll never forget it. I'd already started working out with Denise's morning exercise show and loved how she showed exercise moves that anyone could do, no matter what their fitness level. She also shared a lot of helpful tips on eating. One of my favorites is 'Eat breakfast like a king, lunch like a queen, and dinner like a pauper.' I was so excited to take a picture with Denise but when I saw it I was so disappointed in myself and how I looked. I was the heaviest I have ever been.

"Meeting Denise made me even more determined to lose weight. I continued to exercise in the mornings and started drinking lots of water and eating more fruits and vegetables. Eventually I joined a gym and started walking several times around my large apartment complex each day. I lost about ten pounds. Several years later, I joined the Weight Watchers at Work program and continued exercising. The weight loss was slow but I finally lost thirty more pounds and am now a size 6 or 8. More importantly, I've maintained my weight by changing my lifestyle to include healthy eating and exercise. If I do cheat one day, I'm right back on track the very next day. I never skip a meal, snack on healthy treats, and don't bring anything in the house that I might binge on. Fruits and vegetables are always within arm's reach.

"Seventeen years after first meeting Denise, I was thrilled to book her on my show once again. We took another picture together. Though Denise was still as bubbly and beautiful as ever, I was finally happier and thinner. It certainly hasn't been easy over the years to lose weight and keep it off. But Denise always emphasizes the need for consistency with exercise, which has been a major factor in me being able to lose the weight and keep it off. I am fifty years old and I look and feel better than I did when I was twenty!"

Wednesday

Welcome to wonderful Wednesday! You've started the week on a fabulous foot and should give yourself a hand for making it to the middle of the workweek. Be proud! You're aiming to be a healthy, fit, and positive person, and those goals are within reach. The weekend is around the corner, so use that as a little extra motivation and incentive to stick with your hard work. Just think how much trimmer you'll be come Friday if you keep up your great eating and exercise habits. Your tummy will be flatter, you may notice a little more leg room in your jeans, and you'll have more energy to enjoy your weekend. So don't stop moving—the best time of your life is just around the corner.

Use those newly toned arms to wave good-bye to old habits! Focus on the new, healthy you!

Today we'll be doing cardio kickboxing. I know some people are intimidated when they hear the word *boxing*, but I promise that you don't have to be Muhammad Ali to kickbox. To make this something you can do no matter your fitness level, I've picked some of the best yet simplest kickboxing moves and turned them into an easy-to-follow program. The result is a twelve-minute workout that's extremely effective at firming up your muscles and torching fat. Although other forms of cardio like walking, running, and the elliptical machine are terrific (and important to reach your goal of twelve miles per week), this workout mixes things up a bit when it comes to cardio. If you do the same exercise routine for days and weeks on end, your body adapts so you get on a plateau. Changing your routine not only prevents boredom, but also moves your muscles in a fresh way—and that means you burn more calories and fat.

This fun, energetic workout will get your heart rate up—another reason you'll burn calories and boost your metabolism with every step, kick, punch, and jump. You'll also be sculpting strong, lean arms and legs. Like all the Daily Dozen workouts, each move does double duty, working not just one part of your body at a time but at least two. For example, the jab targets your upper back and triceps. The hook works your chest and biceps. And when you're kicking, you're not only boosting your heart rate and burning fat right off those legs, but also sculpting your butt and thighs.

The Cardio Kickbox Workout will help increase your stamina and strength, two things that make you look lean and fabulous, and improve your daily life. With stronger arms, you'll be able to carry your groceries or kids more easily. If you need to move that big box in the basement or push aside the couch to

HAVE A HEART!

According to the American Heart Association, heart disease is the number one killer of women. In fact, more women die each year from cardiovascular disease than from all forms of cancer combined! These are grim statistics, but there are things you can do to lower your chances of developing this deadly disease. Besides the healthy diet and exercise you're already doing, you can protect your heart with these steps:

1. Get your blood pressure tested regularly.

2. If you drink alcohol, limit your intake to no more than one drink a day.

3. If you smoke, it's high time to quit this deadly habit!

4. Get your cholesterol checked at regular intervals.

GET BY WITH A LITTLE HELP FROM YOUR FRIENDS

Whether you have a large family (like me) and friends or just a close circle of a few special people, your social ties play an important role in many aspects of your life, including your fitness. Research has shown that friendship not only makes your life more enjoyable but protects your health, too. People who have good mental health and good social relationships tend to be the happiest—and the most fit!

vacuum beneath it, you'll be able to do it yourself (without having to wait for someone else to help). Those may sound like small things, but the feeling of empowerment that you get from them is huge. With stronger legs and better stamina, you won't be winded when climbing a flight of stairs or chasing after your kids. Instead, you'll be zipping up those steps or right past your children—all to their amazement.

Life is a challenge. Realize that and work, every day, to rise up and meet it.

Soon enough, you *are* going to see a difference in your body. Stick with this Daily Dozen plan and your body is going to take shape—a beautiful, strong new shape. You'll see sculpted muscles and reap the added benefits of improved health and a newfound sense of vitality—all in just twelve moves in twelve minutes today!

WEDNESDAY'S CARDIO KICKBOX WORKOUT

The more you sweat, the more fit you'll get!

1. Warm Up

This'll give your metabolism a jump start.

▶ BOB AND WEAVE: Stand with your feet wider than hip-width apart, and your arms bent with hands in fists that hover right around your chin (guard position). Move side-to-side, dipping your butt (as in a squat) and tapping your toes. Using your thighs and buttocks warms up your body quickly because they are larger muscles that demand more oxygen. This burns more calories, too. Time: 30 seconds.

▶ Continue tapping your toes as you alternate punching one arm at a time in front of your body at chest height. Time: 30 seconds.

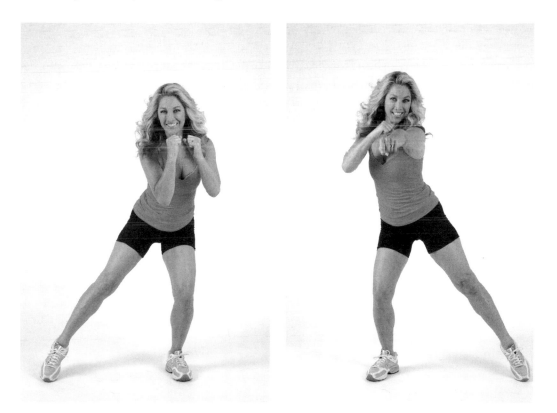

2. Front Kicks
No more jiggling in your inner—or outer—thighs!

▶ KNEE STRIKE: Standing with your feet shoulder-width apart and arms bent with loose fists by your chin, tighten your abs, step forward with your right leg, and lift your left knee to waist height. Continue alternating knees. Time: 30 seconds.

▶ FRONT KICK: From the knee strike, with your knee raised, kick your lower leg forward with your toes pointing up. Your upper body should lean slightly back as you kick. Bring the leg back down to the floor and do a front kick with your right leg. Continue alternating legs. Time: 30 seconds.

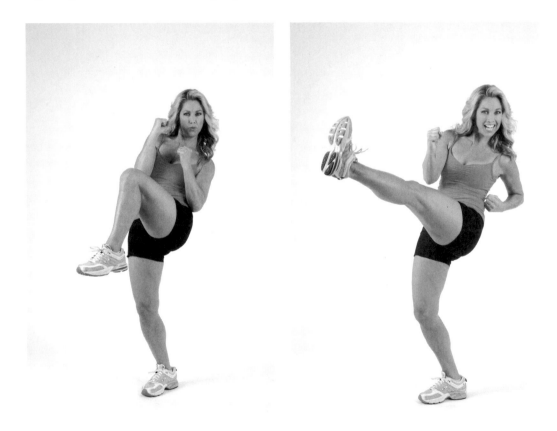

3. Jump Rope

Just think of all the calories you're torching! Get fit fast.

▶ **SIMULATED JUMP ROPE:** Staying light on your feet, do small jumps in place while you circle your arms as if you were circling the jump rope. Time: 1 minute.

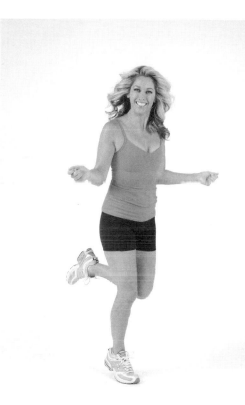

▶ **CHALLENGE:** Jump with both feet together and crisscross your arms in front of your body as you do so.

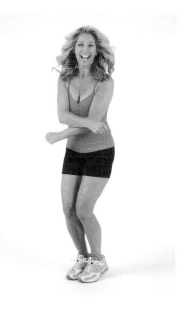

4. Jab and Jack

Create a gorgeous upper back. No more bra overhang!

▸ Stand with your right side facing forward, your knees slightly bent, and your arms bent with fists around your chin (guard position).

▸ Tighten your abs and punch your right arm straight out in front of you at shoulder height (this is called a jab).

▸ Do a jumping jack in the center and then turn your body so that your left side is facing forward. Punch with the left arm, do a jumping jack in the center, and repeat the entire series. Time: 1 minute.

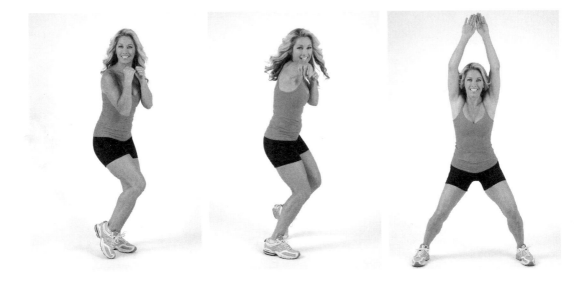

5. Cone Drill

*The lower you go here, the more fat you'll
blast off your hips, thighs, and buttocks.*

▸ Stand with your feet about hip-width apart and your hands on your hips. Step your right leg out to the side about three feet and step your left leg behind you as if you were doing a curtsy. Then step your left leg out to the side and your right leg behind you. Continue alternating. Time: 30 seconds.

▸ As you step the leg behind you, get lower and reach the arm on the same side toward the floor as if you're touching a cone on each side. Time: 30 seconds.

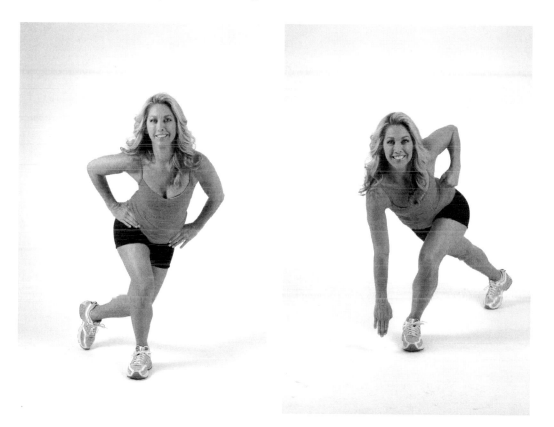

6. Side Kick

Slim your saddlebags with this metabolism-boosting move.

▸ Position your hands in a boxer's stance. Stand with your feet about hip-width apart and squat down low. Keep your abs pulled in.

▸ Step your right leg out to the side about three feet, then bring your left leg to touch it. Step your left foot back out to the side, lift your right leg up, kick it out to the side, and then squat down low again. Time: 30 seconds on the right leg. Switch legs and repeat.

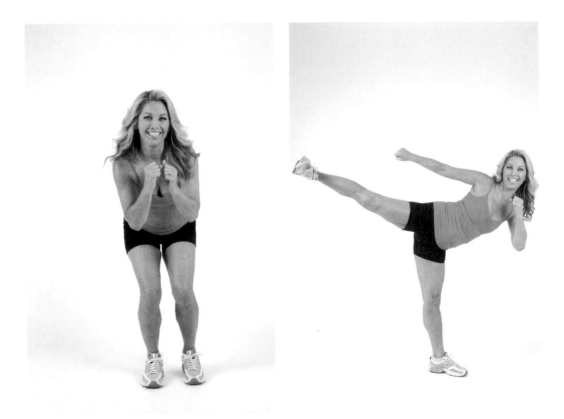

7. Shuffle with Hooks
These punches put sexy shoulders within reach
and accelerate your calorie-burning ability.

▶ Position your hands in a boxer's stance just like in the starting position for the side kicks, with your feet about hip-width apart and squatting down low. Keep your abs pulled in as you shuffle three times to the right.

▶ Stand up out of the squat and punch your bent left arm across the front of your body at chin height (this is called a hook). Shuffle to the left three times and do a hook punch with the right arm. Alternate side-to-side. Time: 1 minute.

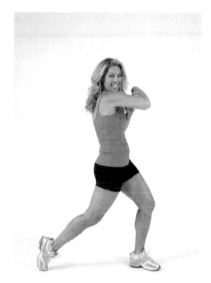

▶ CHALLENGE: Standing in place with your feet wider than hip-width and hands in boxer's stance, alternate doing uppercuts to each side. An uppercut is when you twist your body to one side using your abs and core and punch upward with the opposite arm. Bend your knees and squat down slightly between punches.

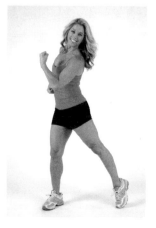

8. Front Kicks, Back Kicks
Kick fat and cellulite far, far away.

▶ Stand with your arms in a boxer's stance. Bend your right knee to hip height and then kick your right leg out in front of you.

▶ Bring the right leg back down and kick your left leg out behind you. If you're just starting out, kick the leg low. As you get more comfortable, kick the leg out higher. Keep your abs engaged (tight) while you kick. Time: 1 minute.

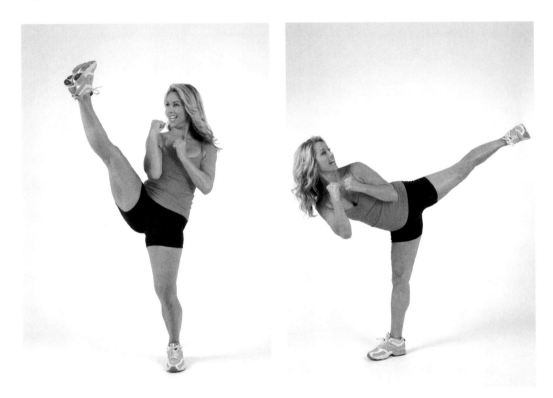

9. Jumping Jacks

These gems from junior-high gym class really work.
Tried and true; proven to blast fat.

▸ Stand with your feet wider than hip-width apart and your hands on your hips. Squat down. Then jump your legs together (landing softly on your joints) and clap as you bring your legs together. Time: 1 minute.

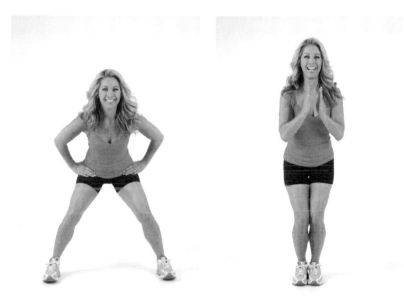

▸ CHALLENGE: Cross your legs rather than just bringing them together.

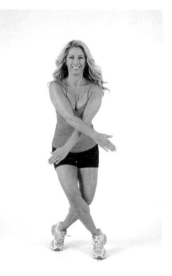

10. Side Lunge

Get an enviable "tight tush" with this lunge. And zap away the fat.

▸ Stand with your feet together and your arms extended straight up toward the ceiling.

▸ Step your right leg out to the side, with your foot facing forward. Lunge down, putting most of your weight into that right leg and hands on your thigh. Push off the right leg, through your heel, and return to standing. Lunge to the left side with the left foot and then return to standing. Alternate side-to-side, maintaining good posture the whole time. Time: 1 minute.

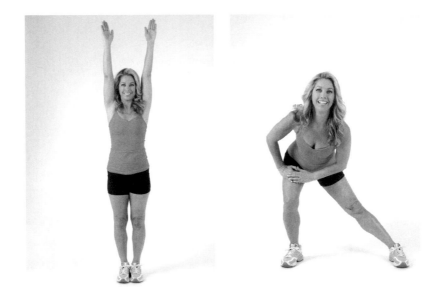

▸ CHALLENGE: Before bringing your lunging leg back to a standing position, lift the leg out to the side, lunge down again, and then return to standing.

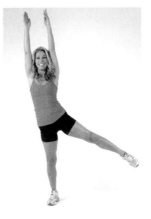

11. Standing Oblique with a Twist
Carve out that sexy waistline you've always wanted.
And keep your metabolism revved up.

▶ With your abs zipped in and back straight, stand with your feet wider than hip-width apart and your arms extended straight toward the ceiling.

▶ Simultaneously lift your right leg off the ground and bend your knee as you pull your left elbow toward it. Then extend your right arm straight toward the ceiling as you bring your left foot back to the ground. Make sure to pull your belly button in as you bring the elbow toward the knee. Time: 30 seconds. Switch legs and repeat.

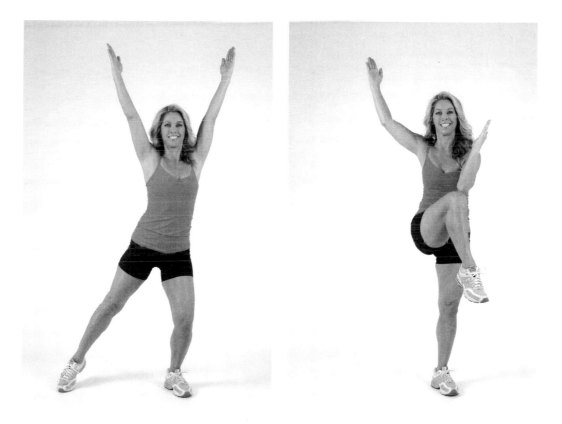

12. Oblique and Core Cool-Down
Target and tone your waistline and trim your torso!

▶ Lie on your left side, balancing on your left elbow and forearm and your left knee. Extend your right leg straight with the foot on the floor, and bend your right arm so your right hand is by your right ear.

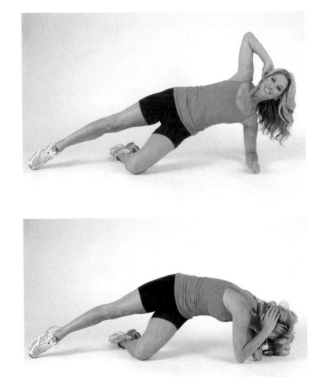

▶ Twist your upper body toward the floor, bringing your right elbow down toward your left hand. Time: 30 seconds. Then switch sides and repeat.

▶ CHALLENGE: Extend both legs straight so you're in a side plank. Twist your upper body toward the floor.

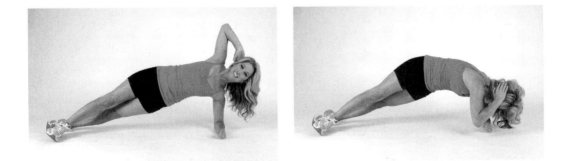

A Dozen Tips from Denise: How to Get a Better Night's Sleep

We're a nation of sleep-deprived people. In fact, a recent survey from the National Sleep Foundation found that 67 percent of women say they have trouble sleeping several times a week. That's a problem for many reasons, the first being your waistline. Research shows that being sleep-deprived can cause you to gain weight—and there may be many reasons for this! Some people think it's hormonal, that lack of sleep keeps our bodies from releasing a hormone that tells us we're full. Others believe that being fatigued packs on the pounds because sometimes when we're tired, we reach for food to give us energy. And on a very basic level, if you're staying up late to watch TV or work, it's easy to eat mindlessly and load up on too many extra calories. Of course, you also need your sleep if you want to have energy to exercise. Naturally, the downside of not getting enough sleep goes beyond not fitting into your favorite jeans or not losing pounds. Without enough sleep, you can negatively impact your memory, ability to concentrate, and reaction time as well as increasing your risk of accidents or injury. By sticking with your Daily Dozen workouts, you're already doing something to enhance your snooze time, since women who exercise regularly tend to sleep better. For a great eight hours of slumber, you can:

1. Do something relaxing before bed. We often hear about the importance of creating bedtime rituals for babies and toddlers, but adults need them, too. It sends a signal to your body that it's time to unwind. Each person has a different idea of what's relaxing, but often it's just a bath, reading a book, or talking quietly with your "honey" or kids.

2. On the other hand, make sure you don't do anything that can get you riled up before bed. That means no watching the news or high-energy or violent television shows or movies (all those disasters and devastation stories are anything but calming). Even paying bills can make it hard to relax.

3. Put away your laptop. "Just one more e-mail . . ." Does that sound familiar? Working on your laptop or BlackBerry in bed can get in the way of your much-needed rest. Besides, do you really want to dream about work?

4. Make it dark. Light causes your body to suppress melatonin, a hormone known to help you fall asleep and stay that way, so start your bedtime ritual by dimming the lights. When it's time to hit the sack, make your bedroom as dark as possible by closing the blinds (get blackout shades if you need to) and turning off any lights. Also make sure to cover lights like those from a plugged-in cell phone, digital clock, or computer, since their brightness can seep through closed eyelids and disrupt your sleep. If you can't block out all the light coming into your room, consider slipping on a sleep mask.

5. Get quiet. Your bedroom should be a quiet sanctuary. But if outside noise or a bed partner who snores keep you up, try blocking sleep-sapping noise with a source of white noise like a fan or air conditioner, a sound machine, or a soothing sound CD; or try earplugs. If your phone tends to ring a lot at night, give friends and family a curfew in terms of how late they can call, or turn off your ringer and let your voice mail do the talking.

6. Go to bed at the same time each night. I've heard lots and lots of sleep experts give this advice. Climbing into bed at the same time each night trains your body to get tired at a certain time, which makes falling asleep a lot easier. (It makes getting up easier, too.)

7. Take notes way before bed. We often have a hundred things (or more) going through our heads at a time, and just because our bodies are ready to sleep doesn't mean our minds stop racing. Whether it's to-dos, worries, or even great ideas on your mind, they can make it hard to get a good night's sleep. If you take a few minutes before bed to write these things down, you'll know they won't be forgotten and you will probably drift off more easily and soundly.

8. Use scents to lull you to sleep. Studies show that certain fragrances like lavender and vanilla are calming and relaxing. If you like either of these aromas, try burning a scented candle and blowing it out just before you go to sleep, rubbing on some lotion, or spritzing your pillow with a room spray just before bed.

9. Believe it or not, your mattress, pillows, and bedding can affect the quality of your sleep. A lumpy old mattress may not support your back or neck, while an overly stiff one can do more harm than good (despite what most people think), *causing* back pain instead of alleviating it. If your pillow is synthetic rather than feather, it may hold five times as much dust mite fecal matter, which can aggravate asthma symptoms. As for your bedding, find something soft and comfortable, and make sure you wash your linens at least once a week.

10. Have a cup of decaffeinated tea. Not only is tea delicious, but routinely making a mug at night may help you unwind. Some teas like chamomile and ginger are believed to be very relaxing and soothing. Brewing, steeping, and sipping your tea can be part of your calming and healthy pre-bed routine.

11. Climb in the tub. Soaking in warm water causes your body temperature to rise. It gradually cools once you get out, and this change in temperature can make you drowsy and send a signal to your brain that it's time to go to sleep. A bath also helps relax your muscles (which probably need a little TLC thanks to your diligent exercise routine).

12. Don't eat too close to bedtime. Heavy meals just before bed can really disrupt your sleep. Since you're following the Daily Dozen Meal Plan, heavy meals are not your problem. However, even eating something healthy too close to bedtime may keep you up. Give yourself a few hours between dinner and when your head hits the pillow.

Sometimes it's not the big temptations that can ruin a diet, but the little ones. You have the power to make good decisions!

Week One Wednesday Daily Dozen Meal Plan

The berries you're eating for breakfast this morning may be small, but the nutritional punch they pack is huge. Blueberries, raspberries, and pomegranates are high in stomach-satisfying fiber and are some of the best sources of anthocyanins, compounds that counteract the negative effects of free radicals—particles that cause damage inside and outside your body. Berries are also believed to help boost your brain power and heart health. For dinner, enjoy this simple Pasta with Fresh Tomato Sauce. I know pasta fell out of favor during the low-carb craze, but it can easily be added to a healthy diet as long as you enjoy the whole wheat variety, which is fiber-rich and more nutritious than traditional pasta. Top it with tomato sauce and you're eating lycopene, an antioxidant with the power to possibly prevent cancer and keep skin looking supple.

TAKE IT DOWN

You know that you should take the stairs instead of the elevator to add more activity to your day. But don't forget to take the stairs on the way *down*, too. One study of hikers in the Alps found that hiking downhill (similar to going down stairs) had unique health benefits—it helped lower blood sugar levels (whereas going uphill lowered cholesterol).

BREAKFAST

1 cup bran flakes cereal (1 grain)

1 cup skim milk (1 protein)

¼ cup blueberries, ¼ cup raspberries, and ¼ cup pomegranate seeds (1 fruit)

LUNCH

1 slice whole-grain bread (1 grain)

1 tablespoon natural peanut butter, for topping (1 healthy fat)

1 tablespoon fruit spread, for topping

1 medium apple (1 fruit)

Men add: 1 slice whole-grain bread and 1 tablespoon natural peanut butter
(1 grain + 1 healthy fat)

AFTERNOON SNACK

1 medium orange (1 fruit)

Men add: 1 medium orange (1 fruit)

1 hard-boiled egg (1 protein)

DINNER

Pasta with Fresh Tomato Sauce (1 grain + 1 protein + 3 veggie)

Pasta with Fresh Tomato Sauce

2 ounces dry whole wheat spaghetti

2 teaspoons olive oil

1 clove garlic, chopped

½ cup chopped celery

1 tablespoon chopped shallots

1 cup roughly chopped plum tomatoes

½ cup low-sodium chicken broth

Salt and pepper, to taste

2 cups fresh spinach

2 tablespoons chopped fresh basil

¼ cup grated Parmesan cheese

Cook the pasta according to the package directions, drain, and put it aside. Heat the oil in a large skillet. Add the garlic, celery, and shallots and cook for 2 to 3 minutes. Add the tomatoes and chicken broth and cook for an additional 10 minutes; season with salt and pepper to taste. Add the fresh spinach one handful at a time and stir. Cook until the spinach is wilted. Add the cooked pasta and toss to combine. Serve topped with basil and Parmesan cheese.

NUTRITION INFORMATION FOR THE DAY:

WOMEN
Calories: 1,270 kcal
Total Fat: 37 g
Saturated Fat: 10 g
Total Carbohydrate: 206 g
Protein: 51 g
Sodium: 1,071 mg
Fiber: 28 g

MEN
Calories: 1,536 kcal
Total Fat: 47 g
Saturated Fat: 12 g
Total Carbohydrate: 245 g
Protein: 60 g
Sodium: 1,294 mg
Fiber: 35 g

DAILY DOZEN TOTALS FOR THE DAY:

WOMEN
3 protein
3 veggie
3 fruit
3 grain
1 healthy fat

MEN
3 protein
3 veggie
4 fruit
4 grain
2 healthy fat

Week Two Wednesday Daily Dozen Meal Plan

It's important to get your fill of fruits since they're loaded with fiber and have natural sugar to satisfy your sweet tooth. Yet I know it's all too easy to fall into the banana or apple rut. This not only gets boring, but also limits the vitamins you're taking in. That's why today's morning snack is chopped pineapple, an exotic treat that's really delicious. Accompanying the roasted pork tenderloin for dinner is quinoa, a true favorite of mine. What makes it unique is that it's one of

PUSH YOURSELF!

Of course there will be days when you don't feel like exercising. So make a deal with yourself that you'll do at least five to ten minutes. Often by the time you get into your workout clothes and start moving around, you'll be reminded how good you feel when you break a sweat, and you won't need much more to keep you going!

the few grains that contains all the essential amino acids, so though it counts as a grain it's also an incredible source of protein. It's a wonderful source of fiber and other vitamins and minerals, too, and a delicious alternative to rice. Plus, you can jazz it up all sorts of ways by using different vegetables, spices, and seasonings.

BREAKFAST
2 whole-grain frozen waffles (toasted) (2 grain)
1 cup mixed berries, for topping (1 fruit)
2 teaspoons honey, for topping

MORNING SNACK
1 cup chopped pineapple (1 fruit)
Men add: ½ nonfat cup cottage cheese and 1 tablespoon almonds (1 protein + 1 healthy fat)

LUNCH
2 slices whole wheat bread (2 grain)
3 ounces roasted turkey breast (1 protein)
½ cup sliced cucumber (½ veggie)
Sliced tomato (½ veggie)
½ cup mixed greens (½ veggie)
Men add: 1 cup mixed greens (1 veggie)
2 tablespoons hummus (½ protein + ¼ healthy fat)

AFTERNOON SNACK
1 medium apple (1 fruit)
1 ounce Cabot 50 percent reduced-fat cheddar cheese (1 protein)

DINNER
4 ounces roasted pork tenderloin prepared with garlic and balsamic vinegar (1 protein)
¾ cup cooked quinoa drizzled with 1 teaspoon olive oil (¾ grain + 1 healthy fat)
6 stalks steamed asparagus (1 veggie)
1 cup steamed broccoli, with lemon pepper seasoning to taste (1 veggie)

NUTRITION INFORMATION FOR THE DAY:

WOMEN	MEN
Calories: 1,283 kcal	*Calories:* 1,628 kcal
Total Fat: 31 g	*Total Fat:* 46 g
Saturated Fat: 9 g	*Saturated Fat:* 10 g
Total Carbohydrate: 163 g	*Total Carbohydrate:* 171 g
Protein: 89 g	*Protein:* 209 g
Sodium: 2,052 mg	*Sodium:* 2,511 mg
Fiber: 25 g	*Fiber:* 45 g

DAILY DOZEN TOTALS FOR THE DAY:

WOMEN	MEN
3½ protein	4½ protein
3½ veggie	4½ veggie
3 fruit	3 fruit
4¾ grain	4¾ grain
1¼ healthy fat	2¼ healthy fat

Week Three Wednesday Daily Dozen Meal Plan

*You can shed your body's most stubborn pounds forever!
Keep going! You'll get there!*

What's on the menu today? One of my favorite smoothies! It's such a quick way to get protein and fiber without having to cook or sit down. When my daughters are busy with school and sports, I love making smoothies for breakfast so that I know they're eating healthy, and starting their day off right. And the variety of items you can toss in that blender or food processor is endless. Today I've chosen antioxidant-rich blueberries and potassium-filled bananas along with vanilla yogurt to give you protein. I also just love this lunch because it debunks the notion that vegetarian meals aren't filling. Idaho potatoes are low in calories and high in fiber, vitamin C, and potassium. Plus, they're so inexpensive! Top your spud with broccoli and you're treating your body to cancer-fighting compounds, too. If you need a pick-me-up come afternoon, the granola bar should do the trick. Just make sure it has under two hundred calories; Kashi and Nature Valley are usually good choices. And then there's dinner, which contains two of the foods nutritionists rave about most: omega-3-rich salmon, which is good for everything from your heart to your hair, and quinoa, that protein-filled grain I've mentioned before.

BREAKFAST
Blueberry-Banana Smoothie
  (3 fruit + ½ protein)
Men add: 1 hard-boiled egg
  (1 protein)

MORNING SNACK
1 red bell pepper, sliced
  (1 veggie)
¼ cup almonds (2 healthy fat)
1 part-skim mozzarella string
  cheese (1 protein)

Blueberry-Banana Smoothie

1 cup frozen blueberries (or strawberries)
1 banana
½ cup nonfat vanilla yogurt
4 fluid ounces orange juice

Add all ingredients to a blender and blend until smooth. If the mixture is too thick, continue to add water to the desired consistency.

LUNCH
1 baked Idaho potato (microwave for 5 minutes or until tender) (1 veggie)
2 tablespoons shredded low-fat cheese (1 protein)
1 cup steamed broccoli (1 veggie)
2 tablespoons salsa

AFTERNOON SNACK
1 granola bar (1 grain)
Men add: 1 medium apple (1 fruit)

DINNER
5 ounces grilled salmon served over 2 cups baby spinach (1½ protein + 2 veggie)
1 cup cooked quinoa (1 grain)

NUTRITION INFORMATION FOR THE DAY:

WOMEN	MEN
Calories: 1,411 kcal	*Calories:* 1,642 kcal
Total Fat: 36 g	*Total Fat:* 48 g
Saturated Fat: 5 g	*Saturated Fat:* 11 g
Total Carbohydrate: 209 g	*Total Carbohydrate:* 230 g
Protein: 81 g	*Protein:* 95 g
Sodium: 755 mg	*Sodium:* 1,039 mg
Fiber: 34 g	*Fiber:* 37 g

DAILY DOZEN TOTALS FOR THE DAY:

WOMEN	MEN
4 protein	5 protein
5 veggie	5 veggie
3 fruit	4 fruit
2 grain	2 grain
2 healthy fat	2 healthy fat

READY, SET, SQUEEZE!

Whether you're working the backs of your thighs, butt, or hips, make sure to squeeze the area at the top of the contraction. Pretend the muscle that you are targeting is a sponge and you're trying to squeeze every last drop of effort out of it. You can do it! And you'll make each exercise more effective!

A Dozen Tips from Denise:
Twelve Ways to Add Flavor to Food

Believe it or not, it is possible to add flavor to your food without adding fat. I've spent years experimenting in the kitchen, and now I have many dishes that are tasty and fresh without fat. They're so good that my husband and daughters eat them and don't really know they're healthy. So skip the margarine and season foods with some of my favorites! These include:

1. Basil

2. Dill

3. Cilantro

4. Oregano

5. Tarragon

6. Ginger

7. Thyme

8. Chopped garlic

9. White wine

10. Balsamic vinegar

11. Fresh lemon, lime, or orange juice

12. Just a teaspoon or two of strongly flavored fats like sesame and olive oils

TWELVE THINGS TO DO WHEN A CRAVING CALLS

Even the most disciplined dieters sometimes can't shake the thought of a certain food. Those stubborn cravings we all get can be more than just annoying. They can derail your hard work and effort! You can get past them, though, without bingeing or racing off track. Here's how!

1. Don't automatically reach for food. Instead, ask yourself if you're really hungry. If you haven't eaten in a while and your energy is low, maybe your body is telling you to eat! In that case, have a healthy snack.

2. One of the best ways to beat cravings is to distract yourself. Take a walk or get up from your desk and move. Sometimes just changing your surroundings can change the way you feel!

3. Do something manual like knitting, typing an e-mail, or giving yourself a manicure. When your hands are busy, it's hard to snack.

4. Thirst can also feel like hunger! Drink a refreshing glass of water and then see how you feel.

5. Sip some tea. With so many great flavors, you can calm any craving. Want something fruity? Try ginger peach. For something spicy, look for vanilla licorice.

6. Call a friend. One who understands what it's like to trim down may be your best bet, but anyone who can help you take your mind off what you're longing for is great.

7. Do your Daily Dozen workout. Again, this will distract you and replace something detrimental, like a potential pig-out, with something healthy.

8. Write in a journal. Cravings can often be more emotional than physical.

9. Take a nap. Sometimes fatigue makes us reach for something unhealthy.

10. Eat one serving of something that calms your craving but isn't full of fat and calories. Crave chocolate? Try a sugar-free fudge pop. Have a sweet tooth? Satisfy it with the delicious and healthy baked apple, which counts as 1 fruit on the Daily Dozen Plan. I've included the recipe on the next page.

11. Pop a piece of gum in your mouth. Sometimes the act of chewing is enough to get your mind off that pesky craving.

12. Go for it. Yes, eat what you crave. But try to have only three bites of it. Savor every bite. Often all you need is a little taste of what you're longing for.

Baked Cinnamon Apple

1 medium apple, cored
Cinnamon, to taste
Cinnamon stick

Preheat the oven to 400 degrees Fahrenheit. Wash the apple. Cut out the center core. Place the apple in a small baking dish and add just enough water to cover ¼ inch of the apple's bottom. Sprinkle with cinnamon, and add the cinnamon stick to the cored center. Bake for 12 minutes, or until the apple can be pierced with a sharp knife.

My Daily Dozen Wednesday Checklist

	WEEK ONE	WEEK TWO	WEEK THREE
I ate my Daily Dozen Foods			
VEGGIE			
VEGGIE			
VEGGIE			
FRUIT			
FRUIT			
FRUIT			
PROTEIN			
PROTEIN			
PROTEIN			
HEALTHY GRAIN			
HEALTHY GRAIN			
HEALTHY FAT			
EIGHT 8-OUNCE GLASSES OF WATER			
I did my Daily Dozen exercises			
I did some of my weekly twelve miles of cardio (write how many miles)			
I did some fidget-cisers today (write how many)			

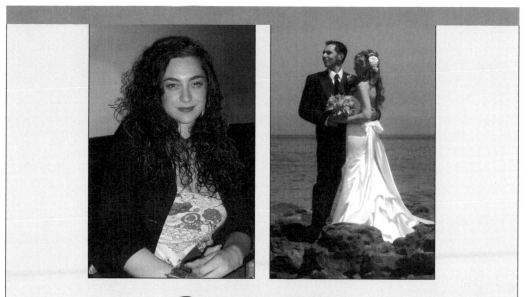

Rosemary Wilhite,
25, sales, Schaumburg, Illinois
POUNDS LOST: 51

As a child, I was thin, active, and actually loved fruits and veggies! I first started to gain weight in college when I was about twenty and in a bad relationship that made me feel bad about myself. I wasn't taking proper care of myself. I would eat very unhealthy foods and I even developed insomnia. I felt really terrible, tired, and a bit depressed all the time. I stopped working out and soon I stopped going out with my friends because I was embarrassed about not taking more control of my life, health, and well-being. By age twenty-three I had gained more than fifty pounds and I didn't feel like I could ever be happy with myself again. That year, I went to a wedding and afterward saw a picture of myself. What really hurt the most was how unhappy I looked in the photo. I was only twenty-three years old, wearing a size fourteen and weighing 171 pounds. I did not want to be this unhappy forever. I'd finally had it!

"I got myself a new pair of gym shoes and workout shorts and began working out with Denise and changing my diet. After just four weeks, I'd dropped two sizes. Within five months, I was down to a size five, and after six months I weighed in at 120 pounds and was a size three juniors—the same size that I was in high school!

"For me, the biggest weight loss challenge was understanding that losing weight is not *just* a diet or *just* working out— it's a lifestyle change. I also learned that the word *diet* does not necessarily mean healthy. You need to change everything, from getting a lot of sleep and eating healthy to working out and having mental well-being and happiness. My whole life is different now. I used to be afraid to go out; now I love to travel, go to the beach, and spend time with friends. Instead of shopping for clothes that will hide my weight, I look for clothes that fit my small frame. I've had people say that I look like a model, and some of my in-laws even jokingly call me Barbie. The best part is when I run into people I haven't seen in a while. The first thing they say is that they barely recognize me; the second thing is that they want to know exactly how I lost the weight. I love it! Now my dream is to do something fitness-related with my life and help others the way that Denise has helped me. I'll continue to work out with Denise because I feel great and have confidence that I never had before!"

Thursday

Happy Thursday! You should feel great about your efforts so far and get psyched up for today's Daily Dozen, an Upper-Body Workout that will give you enviable arms, shoulders, and back muscles. Did you know that this area has more muscles than the lower body? It's true, because the upper body contains much smaller muscles. The good news about this is that when they're worked properly, these little guys respond quite quickly. And there's nothing more motivating than the first time you notice a tiny curve in your bicep or feel a bit of contour in the back of your arm.

There's also nothing sexier and more elegant than a toned upper body. Not only does it look better in so many styles of clothing and create a streamlined silhouette—but it can actually give you an overall trimmer appearance as well. When the muscles of your upper body are more defined, it can camouflage wide hips and a thick waistline by drawing attention above the waist and making you look more proportioned.

In this Daily Dozen Upper-Body Workout, the focus is chiseling gorgeous arms and shoulders and making your chest lifted and your back look beautiful

MAKE EVERY DAY YOUR BEST DAY!

I believe in being optimistic. It truly helps me to shed unnecessary stress. It also enables me to avoid negative emotions that can gobble up so much time and energy. Positive thinking will do more than help you enjoy life to its fullest and inspire your daily workouts. It will also help you bring enthusiasm to everyone around you. A good attitude is contagious!

QUIT THE COMPARISONS

You're one of a kind! No one in the world is exactly like you. It's important to keep this in mind whenever you start spouting gloom and doom about how much longer it's taking you to lose those last ten pounds than your jogging partner, or why your legs aren't shaping up quite like your gym instructor's. Instead of thinking negative, be positive and have more faith in yourself and your hard work! You have your own healthy-weight range, based on your height and metabolic rate, which determines how quickly your body burns calories. Furthermore, different body types respond to exercise in different ways. The last thing you should be doing is comparing yourself with others or obsessing about the number on the scale. Focus on achieving your weight loss goals on your own time line. Do what's right for you, and relish each and every accomplishment!

and toned. These exercises do just that by working these body parts from all angles. You'll notice that in many of the moves, you'll do a few reps and then make a tiny tweak in your form. That's because just a little shift in position can zero in on another muscle group (and area of flab), and that makes all the difference in terms of giving you the results you want. Today, as in all the Daily Dozen workouts, you'll work a different muscle every minute. Like I always say, move those muscles and they'll work miracles on your metabolism! This means you can say bye-bye to flabby biceps, bra overhang, and skin that jiggles under your arm when you wave. These moves also give your chest a boost because they develop your pectoralis major, the muscles sitting just underneath your breast tissue. For women, this creates the appearance of more lifted breasts (no surgery required), and greatly improves posture for men and women. No more slouching or standing hunched over (bad posture is more than unattractive; it can add five to ten pounds to your appearance).

When you just don't think you can, keep going! Getting through those weak moments is how you become stronger!

Today's workout also targets the muscles that run along the fronts of the arms called the biceps, and those that run along the backs of your upper arms called the triceps. One reason I believe it's important to work the triceps is that they're the most underused muscles in the body. In day-to-day life, we use our biceps when we pick up our kids or groceries. But we rarely use the triceps, so we need to give them a little extra attention when we exercise. Other moves in your twelve-minute workout target the upper, middle, and lower back as well as the chest and shoulders. Just make sure to keep your belly button pulled in and tight while doing these exercises and you'll not only protect your back but also give your abs a good workout.

> ## TRICK YOUR EYES— AND YOUR STOMACH!
>
> At meals, take a smaller portion of the main course and then load the rest of your plate with lots of vegetables. Your eyes still see a full plate—even though there will be fewer calories on it—so you will still feel satisfied.

Remember that your form is important and it's the quality of the exercise, not the quantity, that will give you the body you're striving for. Always keep your muscles relaxed as you raise and lower your arms during the different exercises. Keep your neck nice and long, with your shoulders low and away from your ears. Never tense your neck and shoulders. And remember to smile. These simple steps will keep you feeling great. And you are worth it, so pay attention to the details. With your future flat tummy in mind, I've also added some extra ab exercises that work both the lower and upper areas of your abdominal muscles. Do them right and I promise you'll see results.

THURSDAY'S UPPER-BODY AND AB WORKOUT

*It's time to get our weights to target-tone our arms,
uplift our chests, shape our shoulders, and sculpt our backs.*

1. Warm Up

*This opens all the muscles that we'll be working today.
Remember, oxygen equals energy—so breathe.*

▶ SHOULDER ROLLS: Stand with your feet wider than hip-width apart and bend your left arm as you circle your left shoulder back. Simultaneously lean to the left and bend your left leg. Then shift your weight to the right, slightly bend your right leg, and roll your right shoulder back. Time: 20 seconds.

▶ BACK AND CHEST STRETCH: Standing with your feet shoulder-width apart, stretch your arms back behind you as you open up your chest and lean back. Time: 20 seconds.

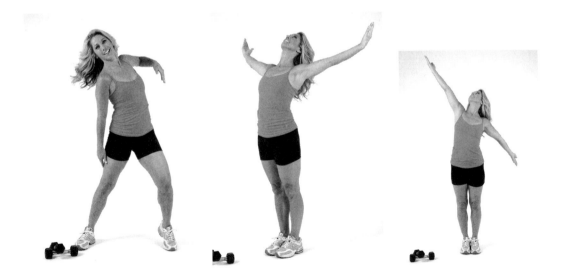

▶ DIAGONAL REACH: Stand with your feet together and extend your right arm up toward the ceiling on a diagonal while you extend your left arm down toward the ground on a diagonal. Lean back slightly and then switch arms so your right is going toward the ceiling and your left toward the floor. Time: 20 seconds.

2. Rows

This sculpts sexy back muscles and improves your posture.

▸ Step your left foot out to the side about three to four feet and bend your left knee. Keep your right leg straight behind you. Rest your left hand on your left thigh. Holding both dumbbells in your right hand, extend your arm straight toward the floor with your palm facing your body.

▸ Bend your right arm and drive your elbow back as you lift your arm as high as you can. Return to the start. Time: 30 seconds on each arm.

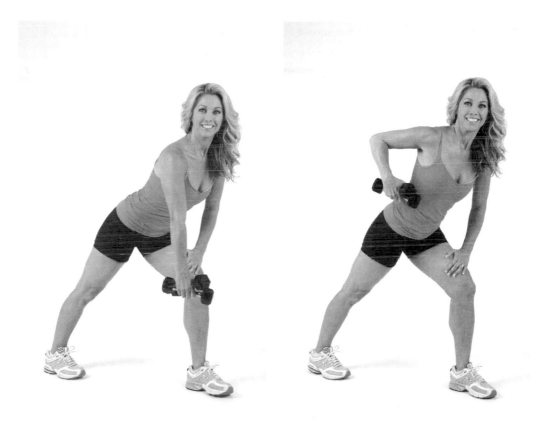

3. Bicep Curls with Tweaks

*Tiny tweaks in your hand position mean you hit all the areas
of the biceps for beautiful, chiseled arms.*

▸ Stand with your feet together and knees slightly bent. With a dumbbell in each
hand and palms facing forward, extend your arms straight down in front of your
body.

▸ Lift your arms up toward your shoulders. Return to the start. Maintain good
posture and pull your abs in as you lift. Time: 30 seconds.

▸ Continue bicep curls, but turn your hands so your palms are facing each other
for hammer curls. Time: 30 seconds.

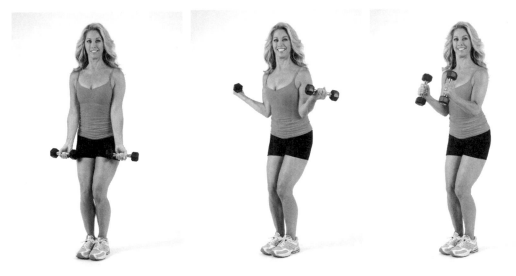

4. Shoulders Medial Delts
Think defined, movie-star shoulders.

▶ FRONT RAISES: Stand with your feet together and knees slightly bent. Hold a dumbbell in each hand with your arms extended straight down in front of your body. Lift one arm up to shoulder height and then return to the start before lifting the other arm. Continue alternating. Time: 30 seconds.

▶ CHALLENGE: Lift both arms at the same time.

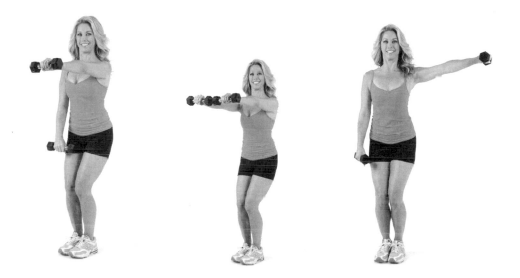

▶ LATERAL RAISES: Alternate lifting your arms out to the side to shoulder height. Time: 30 seconds.

▶ CHALLENGE: Lift one arm out to the side and one arm in front at the same time. Alternate which arm goes in front and which goes to the side. You can also try lifting your arms out to the sides on a diagonal so they look like a V.

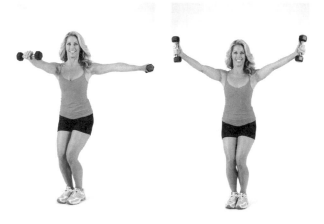

5. Tricep Extensions
No more under-arm flab, no more under-arm sag—we'll firm it right up!

▶ Step your left foot out to the side about three to four feet and bend your left knee. Keep your right leg straight behind you. Rest your left hand on your left thigh.

▶ Holding both dumbbells in your right hand and with your palms facing your body, extend your right arm straight behind you as high as you can. Bend your forearm in toward your body, making sure to keep your elbow lifted as high as you can. Time: 30 seconds on each arm.

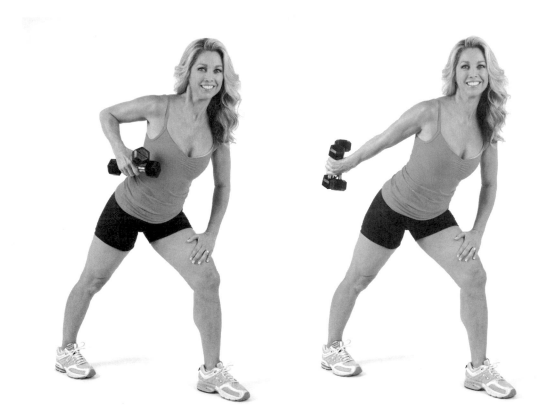

6. Posterior Delts

*Really work that back by squeezing your shoulder blades
together when you lift the weights up.*

▶ Stand with your feet together and hold a dumbbell in each hand. Bend your knees slightly and lean your upper body forward, keeping your back straight. Keeping your elbows slightly bent, extend your arms down toward the floor with the palms facing each other. You should feel as if you're hugging a large beach ball.

▶ Lift your arms up and straight out to the sides. Return to the start position. Time: 1 minute.

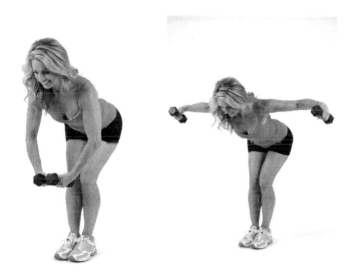

▶ CHALLENGE: Lift your arms, leading with your elbows.

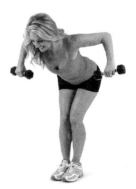

7. Push-Ups

This classic exercise works your whole body, especially your chest.
The staggered hand position targets muscles you didn't even know you had.

▸ Get into a push-up position where you're balancing on your knees and hands. Make sure your hands are right beneath your shoulders and that your body forms one long line from your head to your toes. Also, be sure you're not balancing on your kneecaps, and keep your back straight.

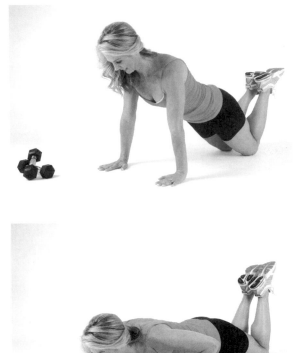

▸ Lower your body toward the floor. Push up to return to the start. Time: 15 seconds.

▸ Position your hands on the floor with thumbs and pointer fingers touching. Then do push-ups. Time: 15 seconds.

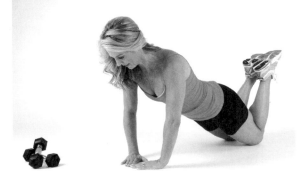

▶ Bring your arms close to the sides of the body for tricep push-ups. Time: 15 seconds.

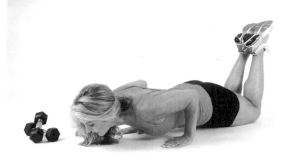

▶ ULTIMATE SPIDER-MAN PUSH-UP: Do push-ups—and each time you come up, bring one knee toward your chest. Time: 15 seconds.

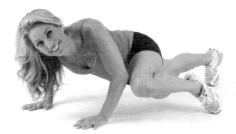

▶ CHALLENGE: Do push-ups on your toes instead of your knees.

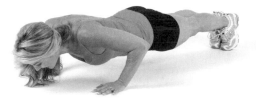

8. Plank Rows

Buff your back and flatten your tummy all at the same time.

▸ Hold a dumbbell in each hand and position yourself on your hands and knees. Bend your left elbow, bringing the arm up alongside your body. Time: 30 seconds on each side.

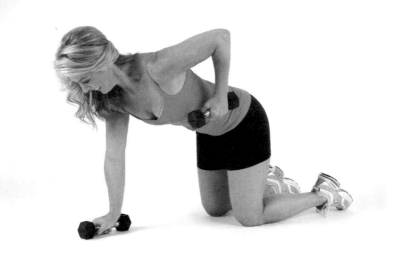

▸ CHALLENGE: Do this move on your toes.

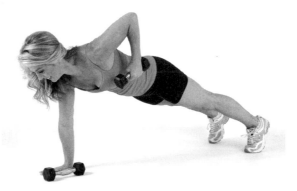

9. Side Plank
Create an hourglass shape and prevent back pain.

▸ Sit on the floor with your right knee bent in front of you and your left leg extended out to your left side. Place your right hand on the floor.

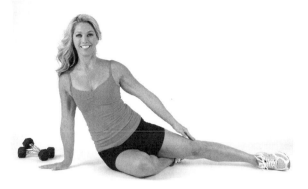

▸ Lift your body all the way off the floor so you're balancing on the side of your right knee and hand. Extend your left arm straight up toward the ceiling. Time: 30 seconds on each side.

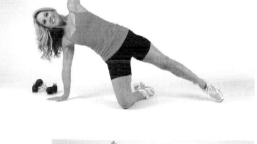

▸ CHALLENGE: Straighten your legs and balance on your feet.

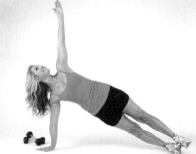

10. Back Strengthener

Your spine is your lifeline; keep it healthy and strong.

▸ Holding a dumbbell in each hand, lie on the floor on your stomach with your legs extended straight and your arms out to the side.

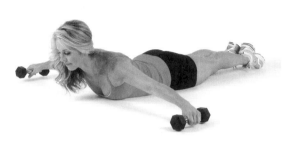

▸ Slowly lift your arms and upper body off the floor, and lower yourself back down. Take your time, making the muscle do the work, not momentum, and be sure to squeeze your buttocks to protect your lower back. Time: 1 minute.

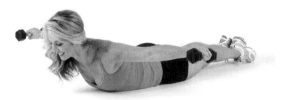

▸ CHALLENGE: Lift your legs off the floor, too, and extend your arms along the sides of your body.

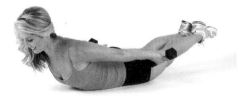

11. Lat Pull-Down with Abs

Flatten and firm your lower tummy and your back.

▸ Lie on your back with your knees bent, feet flat on the floor. Hold one weight in both hands and extend your arms straight above your head.

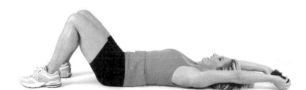

▸ Lift one knee toward your chest as you lift the arms so they're extended right above your chest. Then lower leg and arms to start and switch legs. Alternate legs repeatedly. Time: 1 minute.

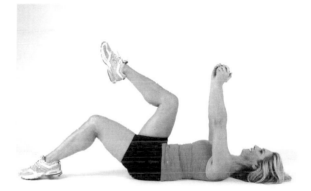

▸ CHALLENGE: Lie on the floor with your legs extended straight up toward the ceiling. Lower one leg as you lower the arms toward the floor.

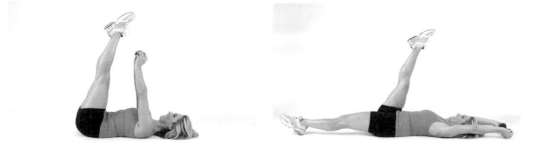

12. Classic Crunch

This oldie but goodie really works. Try all three ways to see results quickly.

▸ Lie on your back on the floor with your legs bent and feet flat on the floor. Place your hands behind your head and use your abs to help lift your head, neck, and shoulders off the floor, and then relax. Lift and lower (crunch). Time: 20 seconds.

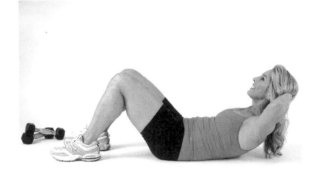

▸ Cross your arms in front of your chest while crunching. Time: 20 seconds.

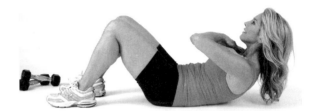

▸ Extend your arms up above your head while crunching. Time: 20 seconds.

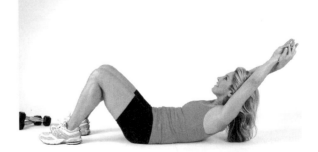

A Dozen Tips from Denise:
How to Soothe Muscle Soreness

With my warm-ups and stretches, you'll move in a certain sequence that helps prevent soreness. That said, muscle soreness after the first few days of exercise is totally normal. (Note that this overall feeling in your body and muscles is different from pain. If you experience elevated pain in one localized area for more than four days, get it checked out by your health-care professional.) Soreness is a sign that you worked muscles that haven't been worked in a while. If you're stiff or sore after your first few workouts, try some of these easy solutions to get you back on your feet and feeling better. But don't quit! Consistency is the key to success. Remember your goals and the reasons you wanted to make positive changes. Then treat your tired muscles with . . .

1. Ice packs.

2. Warm compresses.

3. A heating pad.

4. Over-the-counter pain relievers.

5. A soak in bathwater with Epsom salts.

6. Stretches to boost circulation, which heals your body (see Sunday's Yoga Stretch Workout on page 259).

7. A yoga class.

8. A massage to help release lactic acid buildup, which causes that sore feeling.

9. Topical creams that contain menthol and/or camphor.

10. Lots of water to help flush lactic acid out of the muscles.

11. Enough sleep.

12. Movement. Walking it off can really help.

It may sound contradictory, but research shows the best remedy for exercise-induced soreness is to keep moving. By going for a walk or bike ride, you'll pump nutrients to your muscles and help speed up the healing process.

Eating right isn't about willpower.
It's about changing those bad habits.

Week One Thursday Daily Dozen Meal Plan

Adding flaxseed to your meals is a simple way to get your fill of all-important omega-3 fatty acids. I love flaxseed on oatmeal—like you'll have today for breakfast—but also enjoy sprinkling it on top of yogurt, cold cereal, or salads, and even stirring it into smoothies. You can also mix it into the batter when baking low-fat muffins or breads to give them a nutritional boost. (Your husband and kids won't know the difference!) You'll also have half an apple for breakfast and will want to save the other half to add to your Turkey & Apple Pita for lunch. The Veggie Quesadilla for dinner is proof that you can have food that tastes like takeout without all the fat, grease, and calories. It's a simple, quick vegetarian meal that even meat lovers will enjoy.

BREAKFAST
1 cup cooked oatmeal (prepared with 1 cup skim milk) (1 grain + 1 protein + 1 healthy fat)
2 tablespoons ground flaxseed, for topping (1 healthy fat)
½ Granny Smith apple, for topping (½ fruit)
Men add: 1 whole Granny Smith apple (1 fruit)

BEWARE OF THE SALTSHAKER

Once you start reading food labels, you'll be amazed at how much salt is hiding in certain foods. This can be a problem if you're trying to lower your blood pressure. (Too much can also cause bloating.) For example, salt (and sugar, too) is often increased in low-fat items to make up for the lack of flavor. Pass on foods with more than 480 mg of sodium per serving, limit your salt intake to 2,400 mg a day, gradually cutting it all the way to 1,800 per day.

MORNING SNACK

1 medium orange (1 fruit)

Men add: ½ cup low-fat cottage cheese and 1 ounce pistachios (1 protein + 1 healthy fat)

LUNCH

Turkey & Apple Pita (1 grain + 1 protein + 1 veggie + ½ fruit)

AFTERNOON SNACK

1 pear (1 fruit)

Men add: 1 pear (1 fruit)

DINNER

Veggie Quesadilla (1 grain + 2 veggie + 1 protein)

¼ cup salsa

2 tablespoons light sour cream

Turkey & Apple Pita

1 whole wheat pita
1 tablespoon honey mustard
3 ounces roasted turkey breast
1 cup baby spinach
½ Granny Smith apple, sliced

Cut the pita in half so you have two pockets. Add honey mustard and then divide the ingredients between the two pockets to fill them.

Veggie Quesadilla

1 teaspoon olive or canola oil
1 whole wheat tortilla
1 cup packaged broccoli slaw (shredded broccoli and carrots)
½ cup thinly sliced onion
½ cup thinly sliced bell pepper
¼ cup low-fat shredded Monterey Jack cheese

Heat the oil in a skillet over medium heat. Place all the veggies on one side of the tortilla, top with cheese, and gently fold in half. Transfer the filled tortilla to the skillet and cook for 2 to 3 minutes per side (pressing down on it with a spatula) until the cheese is melted.

NUTRITION INFORMATION FOR THE DAY:

WOMEN	MEN
Calories: 1,223 kcal	*Calories:* 1,535 kcal
Total Fat: 30 g	*Total Fat:* 43 g
Saturated Fat: 8 g	*Saturated Fat:* 10 g
Total Carbohydrate: 189 g	*Total Carbohydrate:* 232 g
Protein: 56 g	*Protein:* 80 g
Sodium: 1,922 mg	*Sodium:* 2,039 mg
Fiber: 31 g	*Fiber:* 42 g

DAILY DOZEN TOTALS FOR THE DAY:

WOMEN	MEN
3 protein	4 protein
3 veggie	3 veggie
3 fruit	5 fruit
3 grain	3 grain
2 healthy fat	3 healthy fat

Week Two Thursday Daily Dozen Meal Plan

You've been eating the Daily Dozen way for a week and a half now, but don't get discouraged if you're still craving unhealthy foods. It actually takes two to three weeks to reset your eating habits, so don't give up! Your appetite will adjust. In fact, a lot of people say that once they get in the habit of healthy eating, they feel sick when they eat the high-fat foods that they used to love. Enjoy today's easy-to-make smoothie for breakfast. I think smoothies are a great way to eat a nutri-

WATCH OUT FOR WHITE KNUCKLES

If your knuckles are turning white when you lift your dumbbells, stop and reevaluate. You should be holding your weights firmly enough so that you won't drop them, not squeezing them so tightly that your hands begin to hurt. After all, exercise should feel good all over!

tious meal without taking a lot of time, and they're easy to take with you on the go. Plus, with frozen fruits you can enjoy out-of-season sweet produce all year.

BREAKFAST

Pineapple-Berry Smoothie
   (3 fruit + 1 protein)

MORNING SNACK

1 granola bar (no more than
   200 calories) (1 grain)
Men add: 1 medium banana
   (1 fruit)

LUNCH

Veggie Sandwich (2 grain +
   1 veggie + 1 healthy fat)

AFTERNOON SNACK

1 hard-boiled egg (1 protein)
Men add: 1 hard-boiled egg
   (1 protein)
1 ounce pretzels

DINNER

4 ounces grilled chicken breast
   (1 protein)
12 stalks steamed asparagus (2 veggie)
2 cups mixed greens (2 veggie)
2 tablespoons light honey mustard salad dressing
Men add: 1 slice whole-grain toast (1 grain)

Pineapple-Berry Smoothie

1 cup frozen mixed berries
1 cup chopped pineapple
1 cup nonfat Greek yogurt
4 fluid ounces orange juice

Add the ingredients to a blender and blend until smooth.

Veggie Sandwich

2 slices whole wheat bread, toasted
1/4 cup diced avocado
1/2 cup chopped grilled or roasted eggplant
1/2 cup chopped roasted red pepper

Spread avocado on each slice of bread, then layer one slice with the eggplant and red pepper. Top with the second slice of bread.

NUTRITION INFORMATION FOR THE DAY:

WOMEN	MEN
Calories: 1,303 kcal	*Calories:* 1,635 kcal
Total Fat: 33 g	*Total Fat:* 41 g
Saturated Fat: 6 g	*Saturated Fat:* 8 g
Total Carbohydrate: 184 g	*Total Carbohydrate:* 239 g
Protein: 76 g	*Protein:* 92 g
Sodium: 1,201 mg	*Sodium:* 1,440 mg
Fiber: 27 g	*Fiber:* 37 g

DAILY DOZEN TOTALS FOR THE DAY:

WOMEN	MEN
3 protein	4 protein
5 veggie	5 veggie
3 fruit	4 fruit
3 grain	4 grain
1 healthy fat	1 healthy fat

Week Three Thursday Daily Dozen Meal Plan

Some people dream about success; others wake up and work at it. You can make healthy eating and weight loss a reality. Just do it!

What they say about breakfast is true. It really *is* the most important meal of the day! Breakfast is your time to refuel after a long night of not eating; it also packs the nutrients and energy you need to take on the day and it helps jump-start your metabolism! I know if I miss breakfast for some reason, I feel tired and sluggish the rest of the day. In fact, studies show that kids who eat breakfast actually do better in school—so think of how this AM meal can help *you* function better throughout your day, too! The best bet is a morning meal that contains protein and fiber like today's whole-grain cereal (one of my favorites is Kashi Heart to Heart) and skim milk (yes, a cup of milk can have eight grams of protein). This combination will keep your stomach from growling and give you long-lasting energy. If you do get hungry midmorning, the peanut butter and celery combo is satisfying without sabotaging your diet. For lunch, you'll have soup—a meal that's always filling. Just make sure your soup is low in sodium and broth-based like today's minestrone rather than a cream-based soup, which can be high in fat and calories. The broccoli you'll eat with your soup is full of cancer-fighting, energy-boosting compounds, and even the little bit of lemon that you'll squirt it with offers you vitamin C, among other health benefits. All my sisters are fabulous cooks, and tonight you'll see that when you taste my sister Kristine's Go-To Chicken for dinner. It's so simple to make and doesn't require any fancy ingredients, yet it has a unique, delicious taste that you'll love.

BREAKFAST

1 cup whole-grain cereal (1 grain)

Men add: ½ cup whole-grain cereal (½ grain)

1 cup skim milk (1 protein)

1 cup mixed berries (1 fruit)

1 teaspoon ground flaxseed

SIP AND STAY HYDRATED

Water is always the best beverage choice, so drink plenty before and after you work out. If you need something with a little more substance to keep you going, try a glass of skim milk. It has the nutrients you need, but it doesn't have all the sugar you'll find in those fluorescent-colored energy drinks. Now, that's the way to hydrate!

MORNING SNACK

2 tablespoons natural peanut butter (1 healthy fat)

10 celery sticks (1 veggie)

Men add: ¼ cup raisins (1 fruit)

LUNCH

2 cups low-sodium minestrone soup (canned or homemade) (2 veggie +
    1 protein)

1 cup steamed broccoli with fresh-squeezed lemon juice (1 veggie)

1 medium apple (1 fruit)

AFTERNOON SNACK

1 cup sliced strawberries (1 fruit)

1 teaspoon brown sugar, for topping

1 tablespoon part-skim ricotta cheese, for topping

DINNER

Kristine's Go-To Chicken (1 protein + 1 veggie)

1 cup cooked brown rice (1 grain)

Kristine's Go-To Chicken

1 tablespoon olive oil

4 ounces chicken breast

1 clove garlic, chopped

¼ cup chopped scallions

¼ cup chopped celery

¼ cup chopped carrots

¼ cup chopped fresh parsley

1 bay leaf

½ cup low-sodium chicken broth

Heat the oil in a skillet over medium-high heat. Add the chicken breast and brown on both sides. Add the garlic, scallions, celery, carrots, parsley, and bay leaf and sauté for 2 to 3 minutes. Add the chicken broth, reduce the heat, and simmer for 20 minutes until the chicken is cooked through.

NUTRITION INFORMATION FOR THE DAY:

WOMEN

Calories: 1,445 kcal

Total Fat: 42 g

Saturated Fat: 8 g

Total Carbohydrate: 202 g

Protein: 78 g

Sodium: 1,670 mg

Fiber: 38 g

MEN

Calories: 1,684 kcal

Total Fat: 44 g

Saturated Fat: 8 g

Total Carbohydrate: 259 g

Protein: 85 g

Sodium: 1,739 mg

Fiber: 48 g

DAILY DOZEN TOTALS FOR THE DAY:

WOMEN

3 protein

5 veggie

3 fruit

2 grain

1 healthy fat

MEN

3 protein

5 veggie

4 fruit

2½ grain

1 healthy fat

A Dozen Tips from Denise:
Healthy and Happy Food Shopping

Your local supermarket is full of tempting but high-fat goodies, thriving under the guise of being a healthy choice. But you can thwart their efforts by being a savvy shopper. Here's how.

1. Never shop when you're hungry. Every tempting food will call your name and climb into your grocery cart. Plus, a growling stomach may force you to tear into a box of something fattening and high-calorie while you stroll the aisles.

2. Have a healthy meal or afternoon snack before hitting the stores in order to quell cravings and keep those doughnuts, chips, and other goodies from landing in your cart.

3. Plan your weekly menus before leaving the house. This will ensure that you stock up on the foods you need to prepare quick and healthy meals daily. With the right items in the house, healthy eating is a cinch.

4. Always read the Nutrition Facts labels of unfamiliar foods to determine whether or not they fit your diet.

5. If an unhealthy food is even the tiniest bit tempting, don't buy it. After all, you can't eat what you don't have in the house, so avoid the high-fat foods that seduce you late at night. If they're not in the cupboard, you won't hear them call.

6. Always shop with a list and don't stray. Keep a master list of healthy foods on your computer and then just circle what you need. This way high-fat, high-cal, and preservative-filled foods won't follow you home.

7. Shop the perimeter of the store. That's where all the healthy items like produce and dairy are.

8. Avoid the center of the store. That's typically where you'll find processed foods like boxes or bags of cookies, chips, and cakes.

9. Don't let sales, coupons, or specials trick you into buying foods you don't want or need. Just because you can buy five boxes of cake mix for five dollars doesn't mean you should.

10. Stock up on pantry essentials like whole wheat pasta, frozen fruits and veggies, and eggs. Always having these items on hand means a good-for-you meal is just minutes away.

11. Shop solo. If going to the store with your children or husband means you'll come home with a cartful of unhealthy treats, try to hit the stores on your own. This way you won't be guilted into buying foods that no one in your family needs—whether they're watching their waistlines or not.

12. Don't nibble while you shop. If your supermarket has samples of food or cooking demonstrations, keep your mouth moving by chewing a piece of minty gum. This will curtail any desire to pop those tiny but fattening cheese cubes or quiches into your mouth.

TWELVE ESSENTIAL PANTRY ITEMS

The following foods are the edible equivalent of the little black dress—something every woman should have on hand at *all* times. I stock up on them because these foods can be used in an endless number of ways to make simple, tasty meals. But they're also bursting with nutrients like vitamins and antioxidants that are believed to reduce your risk of cancer, heart disease, and other illnesses. What I love is that with these twelve essential pantry items, it's so easy to pull a healthy meal together in a pinch. That way, even if you haven't made it to the store you won't derail your diet. Get ready to stock up!

1. Olive oil. This healthy monounsaturated fat is wonderful on salads, pastas, fish, veggies, and more. Studies reveal that olive oil may help lower bad cholesterol and raise good cholesterol—and as a result reduce your risk of heart disease. Just make sure to keep yours in a dark, cool spot to retain its freshness.

2. Canned tomatoes. I love to toss these with pasta as a simple sauce, mix with chicken, or add to chili. Or I'll top a whole wheat pita with canned tomatoes and sprinkle on low-fat cheese for a simple low-cal pizza.

3. Canned or packaged beans. I'm a big fan of all kinds of beans, including black, kidney, white beans, and lentils. They're high in iron and fiber and add substance to salads, sandwiches, chili, wraps, and tacos. Plus, they've got lots of research behind them. Some studies show that beans may help lower cholesterol and blood sugar; others suggest they may reduce your risk of heart disease.

4. Garlic. There's lots of scientific evidence that points to garlic as a cancer-fighting food thanks to compounds called phytochemicals. And there are hundreds of ways to use garlic. I use it in salad dressings, sautéed veggies, chicken dishes, and soups. Another yummy recipe? Roast it and spread it on whole-grain bread for an enticing appetizer.

5. Quinoa, barley, and couscous. These grains make great side dishes and are a nice change from plain old rice. Bursting with healthy fiber and other nutrients, quinoa, barley, and couscous taste terrific when combined with veggies, dried fruit, or lean protein.

6. Potatoes. Everyone loves this number one veggie, and with good reason. It's filled with fiber and potassium, but it also tastes delicious baked, sautéed, or cut into french fries (make them healthy by baking rather than frying them). Both regular and sweet potatoes can be eaten for any meal or as a satisfying snack.

7. Apples. Their high fiber content makes these fruits a filling snack (and one that's easy to toss in your bag to eat on the go), and some studies suggest the pectin they contain can help you feel full longer. I love slices of apple on salad, eaten with low-fat cheese, or heated in the microwave with a dash of cinnamon (it tastes like apple pie without the fat and calories!).

8. Chicken or vegetable broth. With cans or cartons of these broths in your pantry, you can easily and quickly make soups or sauces or add flavor to rice, barley, cous-cous, quinoa, chicken, or fish. Just make sure to look for the low-sodium variety.

9. Lemons. This little citrus fruit can add zest and a lot of vitamin C to soup, steamed veggies like asparagus and spinach, and fish. You can also squeeze it over chopped fruit or add a dash to hot or cold water or tea for a clean, refreshing drink.

10. Onions. Onions add yummy flavor to almost anything. I use them in salads, veggie dishes, and with chicken and fish. They come in different varieties like Vidalia, red, yellow, and sweet, so experiment to find the one you like best.

11. Oatmeal. You can't go wrong with this nutrient-rich breakfast food. It's filling and warm and can be dressed up so many different ways that you'll never get tired of it. Some of my favorite toppings include dried cranberries, raisins, walnuts, cinnamon, almonds, flaxseed, bananas, and fresh berries.

12. Pasta. Though pasta got pushed aside in the low-carb craze of years past, it actually can be part of your weight loss plan. Opt for the whole wheat variety, which is healthier, and use just a little pasta with a lot of veggies and great olive oil. I do this for a hearty dinner that my whole family loves.

My Daily Dozen Thursday Checklist

	WEEK ONE	WEEK TWO	WEEK THREE
I ate my Daily Dozen Foods			
VEGGIE			
VEGGIE			
VEGGIE			
FRUIT			
FRUIT			
FRUIT			
PROTEIN			
PROTEIN			
PROTEIN			
HEALTHY GRAIN			
HEALTHY GRAIN			
HEALTHY FAT			
EIGHT 8-OUNCE GLASSES OF WATER			
I did my Daily Dozen exercises			
I did some of my weekly twelve miles of cardio (write how many miles)			
I did some fidget-cisers today (write how many)			

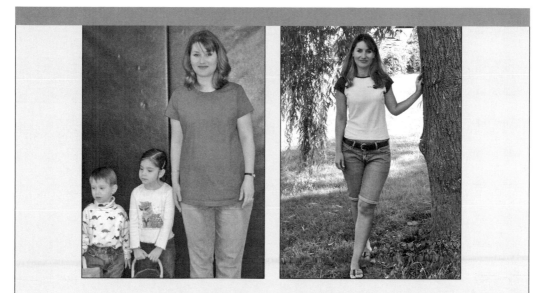

Cheri Lewis,
35, hairstylist and mother of two, Waterloo, New York
POUNDS LOST: 60

I had an extra sixty pounds to lose after my second child was born. I'm proud to say I did just that using the wonderful lessons I learned from Denise. I simply made small changes in my everyday routine. I count my calories (but don't obsess about it), keep junk food out of the house, and take a little time for myself every morning before my boys get up to exercise faithfully—no matter what because consistency is so important. It gets me up and going for the day and it definitely makes me a better person, especially for my family. Because of these habits, I'm in the best shape of my life—both physically and mentally.

"I have also been able to give up my bad habit of snacking on junk food. Now I snack on fruits, vegetables, yogurt, and cheese sticks—healthy foods that give me energy all day long. I've worked hard, but I feel better than ever! I have more energy and more confidence in myself. Anyone really can lose the weight! You really have to want it, and—above all—you must believe in yourself. Anything is possible! Denise has been so inspirational, aiding me in my success. Thanks to her, this has been a life-changing experience! I've realized that the more you work at taking care of yourself, the more you get out of life. It is a great feeling! I'm a happy person because of my life changes and I know that my whole family has benefited! My new healthy life is really worth living!"

Friday

TGIF! Yes, Friday is here and you should give yourself a big pat on the back for making it through the workweek while sticking with your healthy eating and exercise routine. You have put in the hard work and you have made it! You're really doing great. Be proud! Be positive! I know that you can keep it up!

I also know that you're going to love today's Body Boot Camp Workout. It's one of my favorite ways to stay in shape because it works your body from head to toe as it tones muscles, jump-starts your metabolism, and blasts away the pounds. It's a form of interval training where the high-energy segments consist of cardio exercise and the slower-paced segments consist of focused strength-training moves—a very effective combination for reaching your weight loss goals. Why? Because when you're doing the heart-pumping cardio circuits, you're burning fat and calories. Then when you slow down a bit to do the strength moves, you're allowing your heart rate to recover while your muscles keep working. Yet just before your heart rate recovers *too* much, you're back doing a cardio segment again. Then before you know it, you're done with your twelve minutes! With this workout, you'll sculpt gorgeous

ZIP UP YOUR ABS!

Keep your abs tucked in all day long rather than letting them pooch outward. Imagine that you're zipping up a corset, starting at your pelvic bone. As you do this, your tummy pulls in and up. The more often you do this, the more your tummy will stay flat naturally. Do it while you drive, wait on line, or sit at your desk and six-pack abs may be a reality.

CLEAN YOUR WAY SLIM!

Could your house or apartment use a good cleaning? Got a basement or spare room that's packed full of who-knows-what? Well, roll up your sleeves and get to it! Here's why: Housework—such as vacuuming, sweeping, lifting boxes, and gardening—is actually an effective calorie burner! Depending on the types of task, you can burn up to four hundred calories an hour simply by accomplishing household tasks that need to get done anyway. By mowing the lawn, for example, you can burn up to 300 calories per hour; by sweeping, you can hit up to 250 calories per hour. Set aside a time to tackle a project around your living space that needs doing—maybe a closet needs organizing, or you can finally get around to hanging that new shelf—and work away until you finish. Just like that, you've completed your workout for the day, and your home looks and feels more organized! You can't beat that!

muscles, trim fat, and move closer and closer to your goal of being fitter, healthier, and slimmer.

You'll also build muscle endurance while building muscle strength. This is truly training like an athlete and makes the most of every minute, which of course is the goal of the workouts in the Daily Dozen. After all, to reap results in a short amount of time, your workout has to be high-energy, and you've got to both target the muscles and burn fat. Your metabolism will stay high and your body will continue to burn calories and get fit fast. And not only is this workout going to change your body, but it'll help you gain endurance and stamina so you can get through your busy day with energy.

FRIDAY'S BODY BOOT CAMP WORKOUT

If you rest, you'll rust!

1. Warm Up
*Get that blood and oxygen flowing so your body
is ready to blast fat and burn calories!*

▶ Stand on a diagonal facing the right with your legs about two to three feet apart and your right leg in front of the left. With your arms bent as if doing the top part of a bicep curl (which I call muscle arms), lift your bent right leg to chest height.

▶ As you bring the right leg back down to the floor, lift your left leg straight out to the side. Extend your arms laterally at shoulder height. Alternate lifting the knee and extending the leg. Time: 30 seconds on each leg.

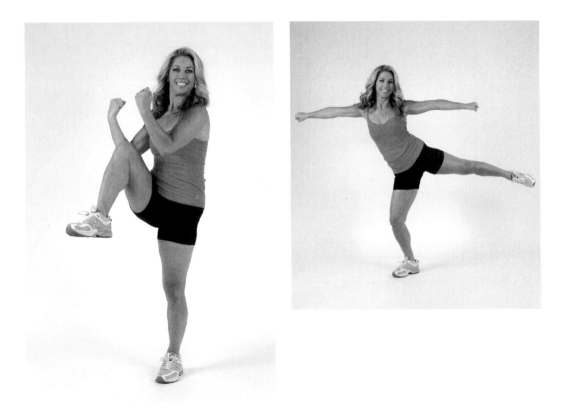

2. Cardio Circuit 1
Slim that waistline! Strengthen that core!

▶ DOUBLE KNEE LIFTS: Stand with your feet hip-width apart. Alternate lifting your knee to hip height two times on each side. Make sure to keep your back straight and your abs pulled in. Time: 1 minute.

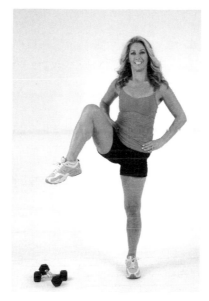

▶ CHALLENGE: Add a bounce and travel as you do the double knee lifts. If you feel really strong, extend your arms behind you in a triceps extension with each knee lift.

Keep your head above your heart as you bend down and pick up your weights.

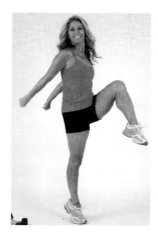

3. Two-Handed Rows
Look beautiful from behind!

▸ ROWS: Stand with your feet together and hold a dumbbell in each hand. Bend your knees slightly and lean your upper body forward, keeping your back straight. Extend your arms down toward the floor on a diagonal with your palms facing each other. Think about good posture and zip up your abs.

▸ Bend your elbows as you pull your arms up along the sides of your body, turn your palms to face the ceiling, and try to bring your shoulder blades together. Time: 30 seconds.

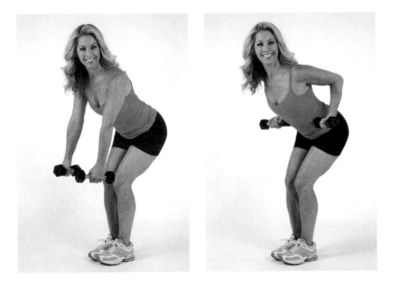

▸ CHALLENGE: As you pull your arms up along the sides of your body, alternate tapping your legs straight behind you.

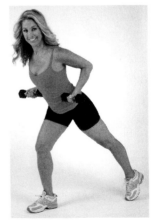

▶ BACK FLY: From the same position as the row, lift your arms out to the sides so they're straight at shoulder height. Squeeze your shoulder blades at the top. Time: 30 seconds.

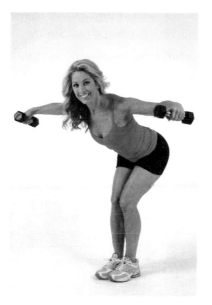

▶ CHALLENGE: Alternate tapping your legs to the sides as you lift your arms. Keep your abs tight and think *Strong core.*

Gently put your weights down and out of the way.

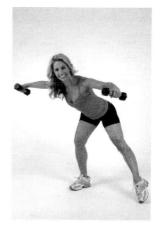

4. Cardio Circuit 2
Burn that fat right off those thighs, arms, and abs.

▶ HEEL DIGS WITH CHEST PRESS: Stand with your feet together and arms bent at shoulder height.

▶ Alternate tapping your heels in front of you with your leg extended almost straight. At the same time, press your arms down. Time: 1 minute.

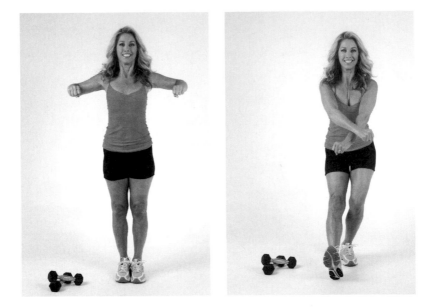

▶ CHALLENGE: Add power by doing a small jump.

Keep your head above your heart as you bend down to get your weights.

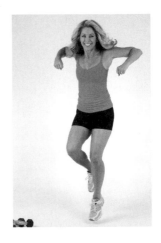

5. Bicep Curls and Lateral Raises
You're creating sleek sexy arms and gorgeous shoulders.

▶ Stand with your feet together. Hold a weight in each hand and extend your arms straight down in front of your body with your palms facing forward. Step-touch your legs from side to side. As you step to each side, alternate lifting the weights toward your shoulders in a bicep curl. Time: 30 seconds.

▶ CHALLENGE: Step-touch your legs as you curl both arms at the same time.

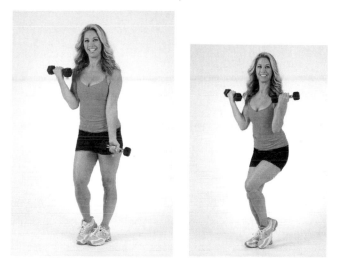

▶ Continue to step-touch but lift the arms out to the sides on a diagonal (so they look like a letter V) with the palms facing each other and thumbs up toward the ceiling. Just a little change works different muscles of the arms and shoulders and really shapes them. Time: 30 seconds.

Gently put your weights down and out of the way.

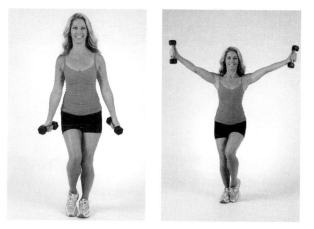

6. Cardio Circuit 3

Think of your body as a fat-burning machine . . . Banish fat!

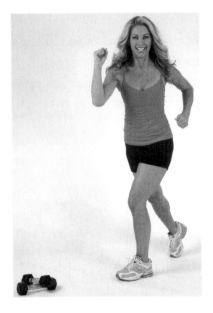

▶ SKI SHUFFLE: Stand with your body on a diagonal facing left. With your abs pulled in, shuffle your legs so that one leg is in front and the other is in back. Bend your arms by your sides and alternate pumping them so it looks like you're cross-country skiing. Time: 1 minute.

▶ CHALLENGE: Power lunge: Position yourself in a lunge facing your left side with your right leg in front and your left in back. Jump up and switch legs so you land in a lunge with the left leg in front and the right in back.

Keep your head above your heart as you go get your weights.

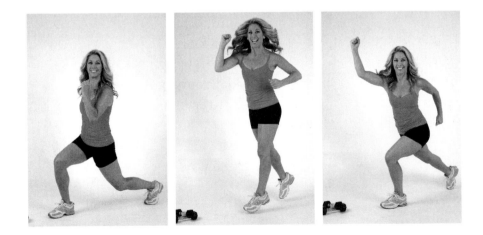

7. Triceps
This is my all-time favorite move to trim fat from the back of the arms.

▶ Stand with your feet shoulder-width apart. Holding your weights in your hands, bend your elbows so that your knuckles are touching in front of your chest. Turn to the right side, tap your left leg straight behind you, and press your left arm straight behind you, squeezing your tricep muscle at the top. Then turn to repeat for the left side. Alternate arms repeatedly. Time: 1 minute.

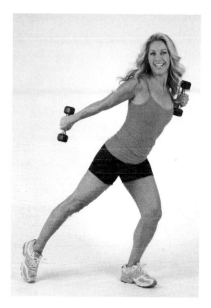

▶ CHALLENGE: Continue the above move, but double it up so that you're pressing both arms behind you at the same time. Also, instead of just tapping your leg behind you, bend down into a slight lunge. Keep your stomach in and your shoulders down.

Gently put your weights down and out of the way.

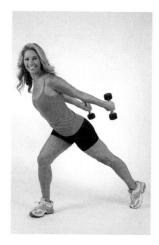

8. Cardio Circuit 4

Work your rear and look as great leaving a room as you do entering!

▶ CHASSÉ: Stand with your feet about three to four feet apart and your arms straight down by your sides. Bending your knees, step your right leg behind your left, as if you're curtsying.

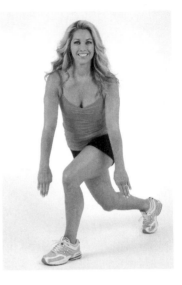

▶ Then step the left leg out to the side, lift your arms up toward the ceiling, and stand on your toes.

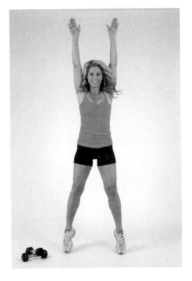

▶ Step your right leg out in front of the left. If this is too hard, simply do grapevines, alternating stepping one leg behind the other from an upright position. Time: 20 seconds.

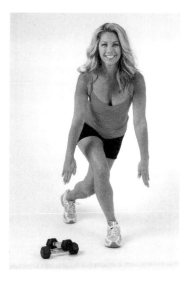

▶ Stand on a diagonal facing the right with your legs about two to three feet apart and your right leg in front of the left. Extend your arms straight overhead and then bring them down in a muscleman position as you lift your bent right leg to chest height. Bring your right leg down and squeeze your rear as you lift your left leg straight out behind you. As you extend the leg, bring your arms down to your sides and swing them straight behind you. After 20 seconds, switch so that your left knee is bending toward your chest and you're lifting your right leg straight behind you. Time: 20 seconds on each leg.

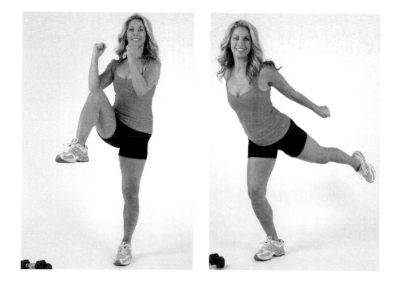

9. Rear Lunge with a Twist
Focus on your core and lift your rear—at the same time!

▸ Stand with your feet shoulder-width apart and arms extended straight in front of your body at chest height with hands clasped together. Step back with your right leg and bend your legs into a lunge position. Make sure your front left leg is in a ninety-degree angle and that your knee is not going over your toes. Keep your abs pulled in and your back straight.

▸ Twist your upper body to the left. Return to standing. Then step back with the left leg and repeat, this time twisting your upper body to the right. Continue alternating legs. Time: 1 minute.

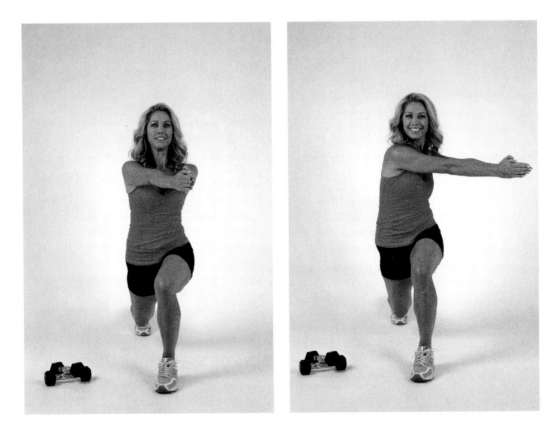

10. Cardio Circuit 5
This is your final cardio interval today. Make it great!

▶ TRIM WALKS: Stepping on your right foot first, walk forward for three steps.

▶ Lift your left knee up, walk backward three steps, and lift your right knee. Now with a little more power: add a little lift, jump to the knee up. Time: 1 minute.

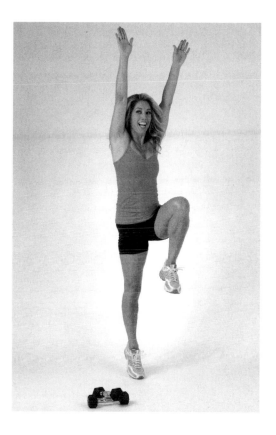

11. Planks

My favorite way to really "zip up those abs" naturally.

▸ Get into a plank position, balancing on your forearms and toes. Hold for 30 seconds.

▸ In the above plank position, keep your abs pulled in and your head in line with your spine so your body forms one long line. Alternate keeping one leg straight and bending the opposite knee to slightly touch the floor. Time: 30 seconds.

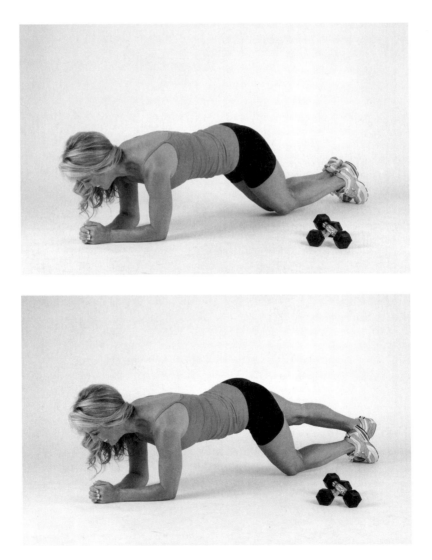

12. Cool Down
Stretching at the end of any workout makes you feel so good.

▶ HAMSTRING, CALF, AND SHOULDER STRETCH: Squat down slightly and extend the right leg straight in front of you with the right heel on the ground and toes pointing up to the ceiling. Stretch your right arm across the front of your body at shoulder height and hold the right elbow with your left hand. Hold for 15 seconds. Switch legs and arms and hold for 15 seconds.

▶ HIP FLEXOR AND QUAD STRETCH: Lunge with the left leg in front, your knee forming a ninety-degree angle, and your right leg extended behind you with the knee slightly bent and foot flat on the floor. Time: 15 seconds. Switch legs and hold for 15 seconds again.

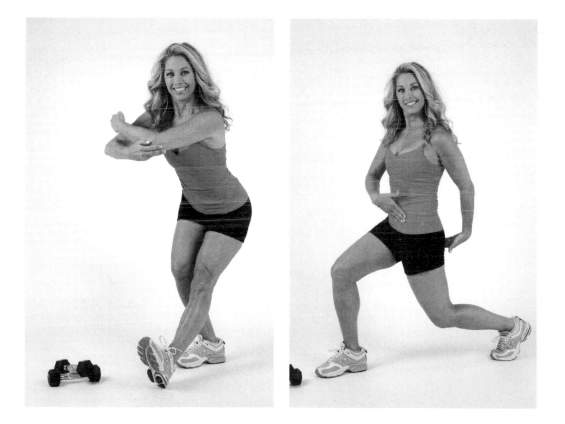

A Dozen Tips from Denise:
Going Green Made Easy

Have you "gone green" yet? There are many easy steps you can take to give back to the environment so we can all continue to enjoy our beautiful planet! Here are a few simple ways you can show our planet your love—and save money and calories, too! Try these suggestions and then come up with more ideas of your own. The possibilities are endless!

1. Carry your own bags. Invest in solid canvas bags you can take with you on your weekly shopping trip so you don't have to use paper or plastic. Some stores even offer a discount if you bring your own bags.

2. Bring your own bottle. Instead of shelling out a dollar or more for a bottle of water at the gym, fill up an aluminum water bottle at the fountain. Keep a mug or glass on your desk at work to refill at the cooler.

3. Pack your lunch. Cut down on restaurant take-out packaging by bringing last night's leftovers for lunch in a washable container. You'll save on calories, fat, and sodium as well!

4. Ride your bike or walk! Save on gas and reduce emissions by biking or walking to work or to run errands. Public transportation is an environmentally friendly option as well. If you must drive, at least combine your errands so you can do them all in one trip. You'll save time, too!

5. Wear a sweater. Turn the heat a few degrees lower in the winter—and a few degrees higher in the summer—to save energy. Stay warm—or cool—by dressing for the season.

6. Sort your garbage. Set aside paper, magazines, aluminum cans, and plastic and glass bottles for recycling. Contact your sanitation department to find out about pickup options or where to drop off the recycling. In many states, you can recycle bottles and cans at local supermarkets—and get back a deposit for each one!

7. Make your own gifts. For birthdays, holidays, and other occasions, create unique gifts at home instead of buying something (typically with disposable packaging) at the store. Bake or cook a special treat, give a nice piece of clothing or jewelry that you haven't worn in a long time, or write a poem on a homemade card—it's really the thought that counts! When my daughters write us letters they are priceless.

8. Let the sun shine in. Throw back the curtains and open the blinds to let the sun in. You'll save electricity and bask in natural light.

9. Turn off the lights. Make a point of turning off the lights when you leave the room and taking plugs out of their sockets when you're not using certain items like cell phone chargers, toasters, computers, and more. Every little bit counts.

10. Shop locally. Buying fruits and veggies from local farmers helps support them and saves money because the produce doesn't have to travel far and wide to reach you. Plus, foods will taste fresher because it's been less time since they were picked.

11. Go organic. When you can, buy organic foods—fewer chemicals are used when they're grown or produced.

12. Buy in bulk. Foods that are available in bulk, such as oats, rice, and barley, use less packaging. Plus, they're typically cheaper!

FRIDAY'S DAILY DOZEN MEAL PLANS

Nothing tastes as good as being fit and trim feels!

Week One Friday Daily Dozen Meal Plan

As a mom, I want my daughters to start their school day with something healthy, so I often make them the breakfast you'll have today: whole wheat toast with natural peanut butter. The good-for-you fats and protein in the peanut butter combined with the carbs in the bread will keep you feeling full and give you the energy you need to power through your morning. Lunch is another fresh take on salad with yummy pecans, pears, and goat cheese. It tastes indulgent but it won't go to your thighs! And I've added a personal favorite to the menu today called Denise's Slim-Trim Treat. It's rice crackers topped with a combination of calcium-rich cottage cheese, tomatoes, carrots, and onions—the ideal snack to tide you over until dinner, which is a mouthwatering combination of grilled shrimp and honey-kissed grilled pineapple. Just wait until you taste a sliver of pineapple with a bite of shrimp. The flavors go together so beautifully.

WALK THIS WAY!

Taking ten thousand steps a day burns approximately three hundred calories and, over time, has been shown to reduce the risk of heart disease and help with the maintenance of a healthy weight. But you don't have to walk all ten thousand at once—and they don't even have to come from what you normally think of as exercise. If you go grocery shopping and walk through the aisles for forty-five minutes, you've walked two thousand steps or so right there! It's easy and exciting to find new ways to rack up more steps! Tracking your steps is easy with a pedometer. Simply attach the pager-like device to your waistband and let it count your steps for you. While there are expensive pedometers with lots of extra features—like a heart rate monitor and radio—you really only need an accurate one, which you can buy for about fifteen dollars at a sports or discount retail store.

BREAKFAST

1 slice whole wheat bread, toasted (1 grain)

2 tablespoons natural peanut butter (1 healthy fat)

1 cup skim milk (1 protein)

LUNCH

Pecan Pear Salad (2 veggie +
1 fruit + 1½ healthy fat +
1 protein)

AFTERNOON SNACK

Denise's Slim-Trim Treat
(1 protein + 1¼ veggie +
1 grain)

DINNER

Grilled Shrimp with Honey-
Kissed Grilled Pineapple
(1½ protein + 1 fruit)

1 cup steamed snow peas (1 veggie)

Men add: 1 cup cooked brown rice (1 grain)

Pecan Pear Salad

Handful European salad mix
2½ ounces goat cheese
1 pear, diced
1 tablespoon dried cranberries (optional)
1 tablespoon store-bought champagne
vinaigrette or your own

Place the greens in a salad bowl. Top with the goat cheese, diced pear, and cranberries; drizzle with dressing and toss.

Denise's Slim-Trim Treat

½ cup nonfat cottage cheese
½ cup chopped beefsteak tomato
½ cup chopped carrot
¼ cup thinly sliced red onion
Black pepper, to taste
6 rice crackers or Sesmark crackers

Combine the cottage cheese and veggies; season with pepper to taste. Serve on crackers.

Grilled Shrimp with Honey-Kissed Grilled Pineapple

1 tablespoon reduced-sodium soy sauce
2 teaspoons honey (or brown sugar), divided
8 jumbo shrimp, raw (peeled and deveined)
1 cup cubed pineapple

Heat the grill or a grill pan over medium heat. In a small bowl, combine the soy sauce and 1 teaspoon of the honey. Pour the mixture over the shrimp and toss to coat. Grill the shrimp for 2 minutes per side or until cooked through. Meanwhile, skewer the pineapple cubes, brush with the remaining teaspoon of honey, and place on the other side of the grill. Cook for approximately 1 minute on each side, or until the juices start to caramelize. Slide the pineapple off the skewers and serve with the shrimp.

NUTRITION INFORMATION FOR THE DAY:

WOMEN	MEN
Calories: 1,243 kcal	*Calories:* 1,471 kcal
Total Fat: 33 g	*Total Fat:* 48 g
Saturated Fat: 7 g	*Saturated Fat:* 10 g
Total Carbohydrate: 167 g	*Total Carbohydrate:* 169 g
Protein: 99 g	*Protein:* 105 g
Sodium: 1,535 mg	*Sodium:* 1,572 mg
Fiber: 24 g	*Fiber:* 25 g

DAILY DOZEN TOTALS FOR THE DAY:

WOMEN	MEN
4½ protein	4½ protein
4¼ veggie	4¼ veggie
2 fruit	2 fruit
2 grain	3 grain
2½ healthy fat	2½ healthy fat

Week Two Friday Daily Dozen Meal Plan

Today's menu contains lots of great grains, which contribute to a slim waistline and healthier heart. Breakfast is a tasty oatmeal and fruit combination so you get your fill of fiber. And I just love this Mediterranean-inspired arugula salad for lunch. It's topped with couscous and lentils—two of my favorites when it comes to protein and fiber—as well as feta. Plus, the simple vinaigrette dressing recipe proves that you can lose weight without eating naked lettuce leaves!

BREAKFAST
1 cup cooked oatmeal (prepared with skim milk) (1 grain + 1 protein)
2 tablespoons ground flaxseed, for topping (1 healthy fat)
⅓ cup raspberries, ⅓ cup blackberries, and ⅓ cup blueberries, for topping
    (1 fruit)

MORNING SNACK
1 pear (1 fruit)
1 cup nonfat yogurt (1 protein)

LUNCH
Couscous, Lentil, and Arugula Salad with Vinaigrette Dressing (3 healthy fat
    + 2 grain + 2½ veggie)

AFTERNOON SNACK
1 tangerine (1 fruit)
Men add: 2 ounces pretzels (1 grain)

READ LABELS CLOSELY

Look for foods that contain at least three grams of fiber per serving and no preservatives or artificial flavoring. For example, my favorite breakfast cereal, Kashi, is all-natural and made from fiber-rich whole grains. It even offers a touch of satisfying protein! Try it with fresh bananas, apples, or berries.

Couscous, Lentil, and Arugula Salad with Vinaigrette Dressing

1/3 cup whole wheat couscous, dry
1/2 cup green or brown dry lentils, rinsed
1 tablespoon olive oil
1 teaspoon lemon juice
1 teaspoon red wine vinegar
1/2 teaspoon mustard
1/2 teaspoon minced garlic
1 teaspoon minced shallots
2 cups arugula with stems pulled off (or mesclun mix)
1/4 cup sliced English cucumber
1/4 cup cherry tomatoes, halved
1 teaspoon crumbled feta cheese

In one pot, bring 2/3 cup of water to a boil. Add the couscous, turn off the heat, cover, and allow to sit for 10 minutes, until the liquid is absorbed. Let cool. In a separate pot, bring 1 cup of water to a boil. Add the rinsed lentils and cook for approximately 15 minutes, or until the lentils are tender. Drain and let cool. Combine the couscous and lentils.

For the Vinaigrette Dressing, blend the olive oil, lemon juice, vinegar, mustard, garlic, and shallots. Reserve about 1 tablespoon of Vinaigrette Dressing, and toss the rest with the greens. Toss the reserved dressing with the couscous and lentil mix, and serve over the greens. Layer on the cucumber, tomatoes, and feta.

CUT YOUR CANCER RISK!

With more than a hundred types of cancer out there, it makes sense to start thinking about what you can do to prevent this disease yourself. Besides making you feel fantastic and helping you maintain a healthy weight, regular exercise may also fight breast, colon, and other cancers and boost your quality of life!

DINNER

Pan-Seared Red Snapper
(1 protein)

Aunt Mimi's Corn & Bean
Salad (1 veggie + 1 healthy
fat)

1 cup cauliflower, steamed
(1 veggie)

Pan-Seared Red Snapper

1 teaspoon olive oil (for skillet)
3 ounces red snapper
Salt and pepper, to taste

Heat an iron skillet or grill over medium heat. Add the oil if you're using a skillet. Sprinkle each side of the red snapper with a pinch of salt and pepper, and cook until cooked all the way through (approximately 4 minutes on each side).

Aunt Mimi's Corn & Bean Salad

¼ cup black beans
½ cup canned corn, drained
½ cup cherry tomatoes
2 teaspoons chopped red onion
2 tablespoons diced avocado
1 tablespoon chopped cilantro
Juice from ½ lime

Mix all the ingredients in a medium bowl, just enough to coat. Serve as a side dish to the red snapper.

DAMAGE CONTROL

If you do binge, use it as a valuable learning experience. Ask yourself why you over-ate. What triggered it? What can you do next time to avoid that situation? At the next meal, just go back to your healthy eating plan. The binge is not the end of the world—it's what you do afterward that really counts!

NUTRITION INFORMATION FOR THE DAY:

WOMEN	MEN
Calories: 1,306 kcal	*Calories:* 1,599 kcal
Total Fat: 27 g	*Total Fat:* 30 g
Saturated Fat: 5 g	*Saturated Fat:* 5 g
Total Carbohydrate: 207 g	*Total Carbohydrate:* 262 g
Protein: 61 g	*Protein:* 77 g
Sodium: 746 mg	*Sodium:* 897 mg
Fiber: 38 g	*Fiber:* 39 g

DAILY DOZEN TOTALS FOR THE DAY:

WOMEN	MEN
3 protein	3 protein
4½ veggie	4½ veggie
3 fruit	3 fruit
3 grain	4 grain
5 healthy fat	5 healthy fat

Week Three Friday Daily Dozen Meal Plan

Eat well 80 percent of the time and enjoy treats 20 percent of the time. It works!

I've heard people say that eating healthy is too expensive. But it's not true. Take today's breakfast, for example. Oatmeal costs pennies per serving, yet it's full of fiber and vitamins. Plus, oats, like other whole grains, contain a compound called beta-glucan that helps your body regulate blood sugar and reduces your risk of diabetes. The walnuts are high in vitamin E, magnesium, protein, fiber, and alpha-linolenic acid, as well as the omega-3 fatty acids that may keep your heart healthy, reduce your risk of depression, and minimize inflammation that can cause wrinkles and acne. Add vitamin-rich fruit like pineapple, mango, and papaya and this breakfast is a disease-fighting powerhouse. For a morning snack,

I love hummus, which provides protein, and baby carrots, which provide fiber. (Sometimes I swap the carrots for other tasty, filling veggies like snap peas or sliced peppers.) By now, you know how much I love beans, so I've tossed them into your lunch salad, along with protein-packed tuna and healthy-fat-filled feta cheese and olives. But forget how nutritious this salad is. It's delicious! Then get ready for make-your-own-pizza night. It's proof that you can enjoy favorite foods and still slim down or maintain your weight. Just find healthy ways to make these dishes and you don't have to give up a thing. When it comes to pizza, I've done the work for you. Though I suggest zucchini and peppers as toppings, other suggestions include broccoli, grilled eggplant, mushrooms, and spinach.

BREAKFAST

1 cup cooked oatmeal, prepared with water (1 grain)
Men add: ½ cup cooked oatmeal (½ grain)
1 tablespoon chopped walnuts (½ healthy fat)
Men add: 1 tablespoon walnuts (½ healthy fat)
1 cup tropical fruit medley (pineapple, mango, papaya) (1 fruit)

MORNING SNACK

¼ cup hummus (1 protein +
   ½ healthy fat)
10 baby carrots (1 veggie)
Men add: 1 cup chopped
   melons (honeydew,
   cantaloupe, watermelon)
   (1 fruit)

LUNCH

Greek Bean Salad (3 protein
   + 1 veggie + 1 healthy fat)
Men add: 3 ounces canned
   tuna, in water (1 protein)
1 medium orange (1 fruit)

Greek Bean Salad

½ cup canned black beans or red kidney
   beans, rinsed and drained
½ cup diced cucumber
5 small cherry tomatoes, halved
2 tablespoons crumbled low-fat feta
1 tablespoon chopped fresh basil
2 tablespoons sliced canned black olives
1 teaspoon olive oil
Salt and pepper, to taste

Place all the ingredients in a bowl and mix to combine.

AFTERNOON SNACK
½ cup Greek yogurt (½ protein)
1 tablespoon chopped walnuts (½ healthy fat)
¼ cup raisins (1 fruit)

DINNER
Garden Veggie Pizza (2 veggie + 1 grain + 1 protein)

Garden Veggie Pizza

1 cup cherry tomatoes
1 tablespoon tomato paste
4–5 fresh basil leaves
1 teaspoon chopped fresh oregano, or ½ teaspoon dried oregano
1 clove garlic
Dash of salt and pepper
¼ pound whole wheat pizza dough
Cornmeal, for dusting
1 ounce fresh mozzarella cheese, thinly sliced
½ cup thinly sliced zucchini
½ cup diced yellow pepper
1 tablespoon grated Parmesan cheese

Preheat the oven to 450 degrees Fahrenheit. In a blender, combine the tomatoes, tomato paste, basil, oregano, garlic, salt, and pepper; blend until smooth. Roll out the pizza dough and place on a baking sheet or pizza stone, dusted with cornmeal. Bake the dough for about 3 minutes or until the bottom begins to crisp. Remove the partially baked crust from the oven, gently flip it over, and top immediately with the tomato mixture, mozzarella, and vegetables. Sprinkle with Parmesan cheese and bake for an additional 12 minutes, until the cheese is melted and bubbly.

NUTRITION INFORMATION FOR THE DAY:

WOMEN	MEN
Calories: 1,403 kcal	*Calories:* 1,678 kcal
Total Fat: 49 g	*Total Fat:* 56 g
Saturated Fat: 13 g	*Saturated Fat:* 13 g
Total Carbohydrate: 205 g	*Total Carbohydrate:* 235 g
Protein: 57 g	*Protein:* 82 g
Sodium: 1,710 mg	*Sodium:* 2,118 mg
Fiber: 34 g	*Fiber:* 38 g

DAILY DOZEN TOTALS FOR THE DAY:

WOMEN	MEN
5½ protein	6½ protein
4 veggie	4 veggie
3 fruit	4 fruit
2 grain	2½ grain
2½ healthy fat	3½ healthy fat

BANISH PMS!

I was amazed when I heard that eating foods rich in calcium and vitamin D may reduce your risk of premenstrual syndrome. Though there's controversy about whether or not you should get your vitamin D from the sun (because of the risk of skin cancer and sun damage), you can get this nutrient from supplements or fortified foods. The latter include cereals, juices, and low-fat dairy.

A Dozen Tips from Denise:
Tips and Tricks for Eating Smarter

Healthy eating is delicious—something I hope you've seen from some of the yummy Daily Dozen meals that you've eaten so far. It can also be easy. All you need to know are a few insider tips that make living a healthier, low-fat, and low-cal life pretty simple. These are tricks I use myself, and they're a huge part of why I've stayed in shape for all these years.

1. Sit down when you eat. It's too easy to forget about the foods that you pop in your mouth while cooking, clearing the table, or standing.

2. Don't eat while you're on the phone, checking e-mail, or watching TV. One study found that people ate an average of over 40 percent more potato chips while watching TV than they did when they weren't tuning in to the tube. That's not surprising, since being distracted means you don't notice what you inhale.

3. Eat slowly. It takes fifteen to twenty minutes after eating for your brain to register that you're full. Eat too fast and you can take in more calories than your body actually wants or needs. Before you take seconds or give in to a giant dessert, wait. If you're still hungry half an hour later, then you truly didn't eat enough and need more food. But chances are that you'll be full. Remember, no one says you have to clean your plate!

4. Write down what you eat. Keeping a food log helps ward off mindless eating and allows you to be more conscious of every morsel. It also keeps you accountable—after all, if you have to write down that you ate that pizza crust off your child's plate or doughnut at a morning meeting, you'll probably think twice. It worked well for women in one study, who lost seven pounds more than participants who didn't jot down their snacks and meals.

5. Don't sip your calories away. It's very easy to forget that certain beverages—like juice, soda, and coffee drinks—have calories because they typically don't leave us feeling full. However, just one 8-ounce soda or juice can have more than a hundred calories, and a frothy, creamy creation from your favorite coffee shop can have hundreds. Your best bet is to stick with water (find ways to jazz it up on page 92). It's calorie-free and, well, free.

6. Sneak filling and fiber-rich produce into your meals (and your family's) by shredding zucchini into pasta sauce, adding mashed sweet potatoes to muffin recipes, and topping homemade pizza with lots of veggies.

7. Stock up on frozen fruits and veggies. I use them all the time, especially when favorites like berries and peaches are out of season. They require minimal preparation—and in terms of nutrients, they can actually be more nutritious than fresh produce that's been sitting at the supermarket too long.

8. Put a curfew on the kitchen. Our bodies need three hours to help metabolize our dinners. Because you're not as active at night, your body isn't burning off the calories like it does during the day when you're active. So if you usually go to bed at 11 PM, try not to eat anything after 8 PM.

9. Don't ban one whole food group from your diet. I'm a big believer in balance. Cutting out a whole universe of food—like desserts, carbs, or fat—has never worked for me. I always wind up craving what I can't have and then I feel like a failure when I cave in. The real key is moderation. Eat what you want, but be mindful of the amounts you are consuming.

10. Serve yourself less. Researchers have figured out that you can eat up to 20 percent less and feel just as satisfied! So when you're serving yourself dinner—or any meal—put about 20 percent less on your plate than you think you'll eat. Most likely, you won't be hungry for any more food.

11. Don't keep the serving plates on the table. Instead, after you fill your plate, put the rest of the food in the kitchen or even pack it away in the refrigerator and *then* sit down to eat. This way you're not picking at food or serving yourself seconds just because it's in front of you.

12. If you're at a party or social gathering, don't stand near the buffet table. And if you're having a drink, have a glass of water before and after that glass of wine.

TWELVE WAYS TO PREVENT BELLY BLOAT

Nothing is more uncomfortable than a distended belly. It makes your clothes fit too snugly—or not at all—and that can really turn your mood sour. Unfortunately, that blue state of mind can be the start of a downward spiral. But there are some simple ways to deflate your midsection and prevent belly bloat in the first place.

1. Eat slowly. Chow down too fast and you can swallow too much air along with your food.

2. Drink lots of water. It sounds contradictory, but drinking water actually helps flush extra fluid from your body. (This is especially helpful during that time of the month.)

3. Steer clear of sugar substitutes. Though it's not exactly clear why these may inflate your belly, avoid them if you can. Not only to keep your stomach flat but also because some studies show that eating low-cal artificial sweeteners actually makes people *gain* weight. Go figure!

4. Don't chew gum. It's believed that you take in too much air when you chew gum, and that can fill your tummy. Also, some gums contain artificial sweeteners that are believed to puff you up.

5. Go easy on the salt. This may sound easy, but even if you don't reach for the salt-shaker, lots of foods have hidden sodium in them. Make sure to read the Nutrition Label to see how much is lurking in your food. The American Heart Association recommends less than twenty-three hundred milligrams (one teaspoon) per day.

6. Don't sip from a straw. As with eating too fast and chomping on gum, you may gulp too much air when you sip from a straw.

7. Avoid too many carbonated beverages. All the bubbles in your glass make their way inside your tummy.

8. Drink mint or ginger teas. These spices are both reputed to help calm a too-full belly (as well as nausea).

9. Sip hot water with a few squeezes of lemon. The hot water and citrus are thought to soothe your stomach.

10. Take a brisk walk or do some other form of cardio exercise. Sometimes just getting physical gets things moving inside your tummy.

11. Try some yoga poses. Like cardio workouts, yoga increases circulation, which can relieve the fluid buildup that causes bloating. One that's believed to help: Lie on your back with your legs extended all the way up a wall.

12. Eat foods that naturally flush water from the body, such as asparagus and grapefruit.

My Daily Dozen Friday Checklist

	WEEK ONE	WEEK TWO	WEEK THREE
I ate my Daily Dozen Foods			
VEGGIE			
VEGGIE			
VEGGIE			
FRUIT			
FRUIT			
FRUIT			
PROTEIN			
PROTEIN			
PROTEIN			
HEALTHY GRAIN			
HEALTHY GRAIN			
HEALTHY FAT			
EIGHT 8-OUNCE GLASSES OF WATER			
I did my Daily Dozen exercises			
I did some of my weekly twelve miles of cardio (write how many miles)			
I did some fidget-cisers today (write how many)			

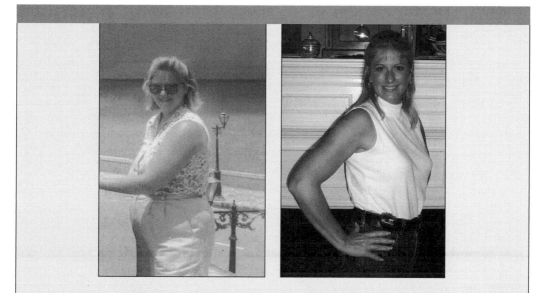

Elizabeth Clark,

37, housewife and aerobics instructor, Olive Branch, Mississippi

POUNDS LOST: 58

When I decided that I wanted to lose weight, I bought Denise's *Hit the Spot: Thighs, Arms,* and *Abs* videos. I had a lot of success with these tapes, but I needed more. So I started taping and doing her *Fit & Lite* and *Daily Workout* shows every day. After finding Denise's website and gaining the friendship, encouragement, and support from all the wonderful people there—I was encouraged to follow one of Denise's three-week programs. I followed it to the letter and lost ten pounds. But even better were the inspirational Deniseologies and the positive energy that I gained every day. I learned that I am worth the time and effort to make myself a better person on the inside as well as the outside.

"Changing my eating habits from soda, fast food, and processed meals doesn't mean I'm 'giving up the good stuff' and depriving myself. I eat what I want, but what I want has now changed. I choose healthier foods and I feel *great*—I'm energetic and satisfied, not tired and stuffed. I don't miss all the junk. Because I feel so good, I'm out there enjoying life, instead of sitting in front of the television and feeling blah. Each month I set goals for myself, and, as a reward for reaching those goals, I buy a new Denise Austin video. I am up to around twenty-five videos so far, and love every one of them. Each one offers a new and different workout. I set a routine each Sunday night for three days of cardio and two days of strength training, with weekends being 'whatever I feel like' days. All of Denise's books give me information in a plain and simple way that I—an everyday mother of three—can understand.

"I recently received my group instructor certificate to teach aerobics and am planning on getting my personal trainer's certificate. My life has changed 180 degrees since I started with Denise Austin. The highlight was when I actually met Denise in person! She is truly as bubbly, sweet, happy, and caring in person as she comes across in her videos, books, and TV shows."

If you recline, you decline. If you sit, you quit. If you don't use it, you will lose it. And we need all the metabolism-boosting muscle we can get.

Saturday

Welcome to the weekend! You deserve to feel good about the work you've put in on this plan so far. Keep it up this weekend and you'll be thrilled at the results you see in the days to come. I know that every little bit of success will help spur you on and motivate you to keep going. It's true that weekends can be tricky when it comes to healthy eating and exercise, because many of us want to relax a bit and our lives are less structured. Rather than work and school, outings may include parties, barbecues, or other food-centered get-togethers. But that's the great thing about the Daily Dozen Plan. It's made to work *with* your life and blend in seamlessly. You don't have to rearrange your schedule to get in your twelve minutes of exercise. Just squeeze it in, do it, and move on. The good thing about this workout is that besides blasting fat and toning you up, it'll give you the energy to enjoy your weekend even more. (Which is one reason I love to do it on a Saturday morning to help jump-start my day!)

Today you'll be doing a really fun Athletic Kettlebell-Inspired Workout. Kettlebells are cast-iron weights that origi-

SOOTHING SERENITY!

Stay mindful during your workout. Try not to allow yourself to think about any of your daily responsibilities—be these work, kids, or the laundry you need to deal with. Your exercise time is your time to just be. Focus on your breathing, your muscles, and your body. Let exercise do the work of meditation and soothe away any stress or tension. Celebrate your body and carry the calmness with you all day long!

nated in Russia. They look sort of like a bowling ball with a handle and have been popular workout tools among serious athletes for decades. However, they've recently made their way into the hands of regular exercisers like you and me. Exercising with kettlebells can boost your endurance, strength, agility, and balance while also giving you an aerobic workout. I've thus taken some of the best moves from a kettlebell workout and tweaked them so that you can do them with the same hand weights that you've been using all along. For this workout, you'll need five-pound weights, or eight pounds if you're more advanced. This is a great introduction to kettlebells and perfect for the beginning or intermediate exerciser. (As you advance, you can always get yourself a pair of kettlebells if you'd like.)

The moves you'll do today strengthen your muscles using controlled momentum. Because of the unique way that you're holding and moving the weights, you're challenging the muscles in a new way. For example, in the double-arm swing you're holding a weight straight out in front of you at chest height and swinging it down and up using controlled momentum. When using kettlebells or your weights, the fulcrum (or pivot point) is different compared with other types of exercise tools, so you're targeting—and challenging—your muscles in a new way. The swinging action also puts traction on the bones and muscles, which is a wonderful way to make them healthy and strong. Not only is this type of movement fun (when else do you actually get to swing weights around?), but you also get a cardio workout along with one that will tone you up. You're strengthening the muscles surrounding your joints with low-impact movements that are neither jumping nor jarring.

Just like the Body Boot Camp Workout you did yesterday, this athletic

Once you get in shape, you'll be amazed at how many other goals you'll want to achieve in your life. Fitness breeds enthusiasm!

kettlebell-inspired routine blends bouts of cardio movement with toning moves so you reap the benefits of interval training. Because you keep moving, it boosts your heart rate up to burn fat and calories, and sculpts and tones all the muscles from head to toe. It's also a form of functional training, which means that you're exercising your body and muscles the way you use them in real life. This makes it easier to do daily activities where you're lifting, carrying, pushing, and pulling, and helps prevent injuries from these movements in your day-to-day life. Just do the best that you can each time you try this fun, athletic workout, and I promise you'll see changes in your body and your life. You'll see success whether it's pounds shed, lower dress size, muscles sculpted, or all of the above! You'll look awesome! I always say that when you finish a workout, you don't simply feel better. You feel better about yourself. Today's workout is proof positive of that. I promise!

THINK BIG PICTURE

In this life, you can't afford to lose sight of the big picture when it comes to your inner and outer beauty. Are you doing all you can to take care of your health? Are you proud of your character and your relationships with your family, friends, and others? Focus more on being a good person and worry less about superficial things. Soon your true beauty will reflect back at you in the mirror.

Raise the bar! Set tiny goals for yourself, and as you meet them, set more. The sky is the limit!

1. Warm Up

Warm up your legs and back while working your abs.

▶ SQUAT REACH: Stand with your feet shoulder-width apart and squat down as if you're sitting in a chair. Extend your arms by your sides but behind you.

▶ Squeeze your buttocks and legs to stand up. As you stand, extend your arms up toward the ceiling and lift your left knee. Swing your arms down toward the ground as you squat. (You'll see that this is one of the fundamental movements in this kettlebell workout.) Alternate lifting your knees. Time: 20 seconds.

▶ WAIST TWIST: Continue to warm up your back and trim and slim your waistline by standing with your feet wider than hip-width. Bend your elbows so your hands are in front of your chest with elbows out to the sides. Keep your abs pulled in as you twist from side to side. Time: 20 seconds.

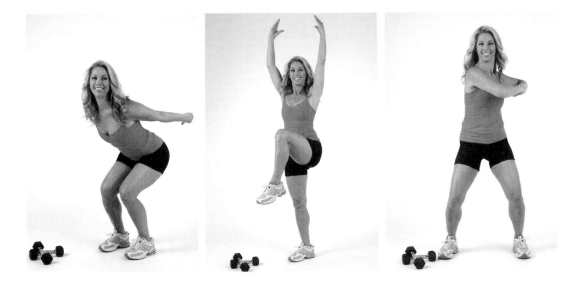

▶ BACK LUNGE: Stand with your feet shoulder-width apart and your arms by your sides. Step backward two to three feet with your left leg and bend your legs into a lunge position. As you lunge, place your hands on your thighs. Return to standing and continue lunging, alternating your legs. Time: 20 seconds.

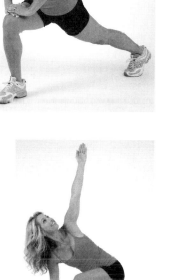

▶ CHALLENGE: When you lunge, extend the arm that's on the same side as the front leg up toward the ceiling and the other arm down toward the floor.

2. Double-Arm Swing

*The power here comes from your hips, thighs,
and buttocks as you reshape your bottom half.*

▶ Stand with your feet wider than hip-width apart and your toes facing slightly outward with a natural turnout. Hold a dumbbell with one hand on either end. Extend your arms straight in front of your body at chest height.

▶ Bend your knees and squat down, placing most of your weight in your heels. As you squat, use control to swing the dumbbell down toward the ground and between your legs. As you return to standing, squeeze your rear, the backs of your legs, and abs, and swing the dumbbell up to right above your head. Your swinging motion should be smooth and fluid, and you should feel a little suspension at the top. Time: 1 minute.

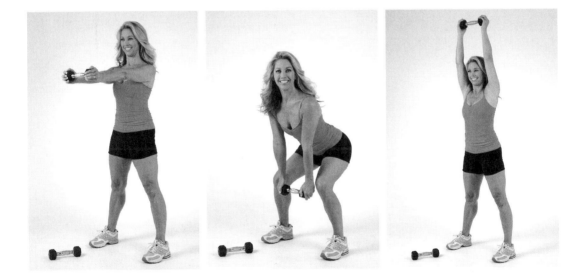

3. Single-Arm Swing/Pull-Back

This is a great way to tone up your legs and upper back and blast fat.
All this in one move!

▸ Get into the same squat position as the double-arm swing, but hold the dumbbell in your right hand with your palm facing the floor and extend your arm straight down in front of you. Keep your left arm by your left side. Squat down with your legs, making sure to keep most of your weight in your heels.

▸ As you stand up, swing your right arm up to shoulder height.

▸ Then pull your right elbow back, as in a row. Time: 30 seconds. Switch arms and repeat.

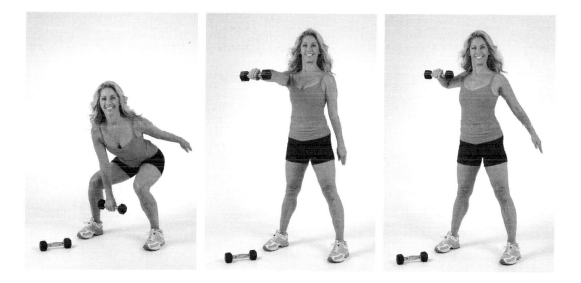

4. Pass-Through

Get your heart rate up and burn fat.

▸ Stand with your feet wider than hip-width apart and your toes turned slightly outward. Hold a dumbbell in your right hand with your arm extended straight down by your side. Bend your legs and squat down.

▸ Bring your left arm behind your left leg and pass the dumbbell through your legs from the right hand to the left. Return to standing. Repeat the squat, this time passing the dumbbell from your left hand through your legs to your right hand. Move the one weight through the legs in a figure-eight motion. Time: 1 minute.

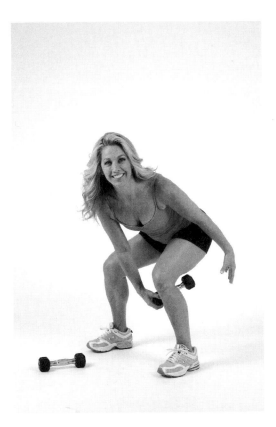

5. The Windmill

This classic kettlebell move trims the sides
of the waistline and sculpts your legs.

▶ Stand with your feet wider than hip-width apart, your left toes facing forward, and your right toes slightly turned out toward the right side. Hold a dumbbell in your left hand and bend your elbow so that the dumbbell is near your shoulder with your palm facing forward. Push your left hip toward the left side as you shift your weight, and your upper body down toward the right.

▶ Reach down your right leg with your right hand. At the same time, straighten your left arm and extend it toward the ceiling. Squeezing your inner thighs as you bring your upper body back to your starting position and shift your weight back, pull your left arm down so the dumbbell is back in front of your shoulder. In addition to your thighs, you should feel this through your waistline and hips. Time: 30 seconds. Switch sides and repeat.

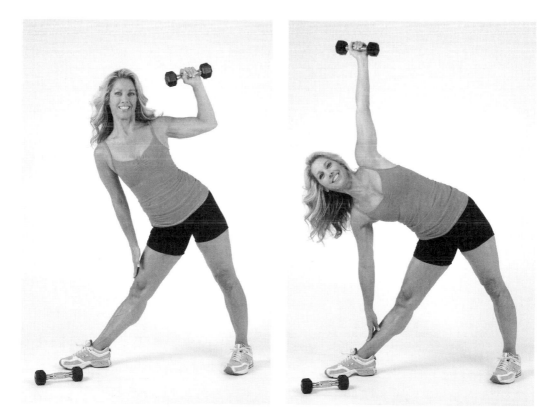

6. One-Leg Squat
You will really feel this in your thighs, and it will zero in on each butt cheek.

▶ Stand with feet hip-width apart and your upper body upright. Hold a weight in front of your chest with both hands. Step your left foot out a few inches in front of your right and resting on your left toes. Lower and lift your body in small pulses, making sure your body's weight is pushing through your right heel. That way you will really feel it in the buns. Time: 10 seconds.

▶ From the above position, bring your slightly bent left leg out to the side, resting on a toe. Pulse down. Time: 10 seconds.

▶ Then bring your left leg back behind you, still resting on a toe, and pulse down. Time: 10 seconds. Switch legs and repeat the entire series of one-leg squats on the other leg.

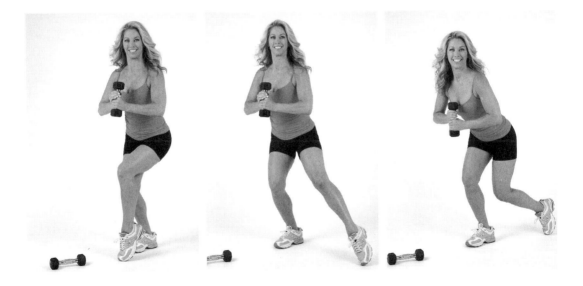

7. Lunge

Imagine yourself looking fabulous in your jeans—from every angle.

▶ Stand with your feet together, arms straight out to the sides at shoulder level, and one weight in your left hand.

▶ Step forward with your left leg and bend your legs so that you're in a lunge. Make sure your front knee is in a ninety-degree angle and that your knee does not go over your toes. As you lunge down, pass the weight under your knee from one hand to the other. Return to standing. Now lunge forward with the right leg. Alternate your legs as you lunge and continue to pass the weight through your legs from hand to hand. Time: 1 minute.

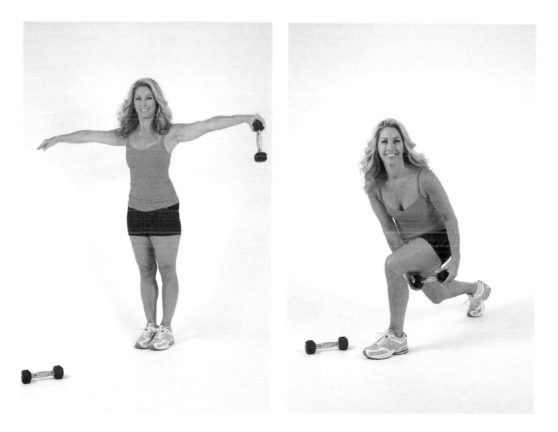

8. Rows and Triceps

Look gorgeous in those sleeveless blouses.

▸ Stand with your feet together and hold a dumbbell in each hand.

▸ Bend your knees slightly and lean your upper body forward, keeping your back straight. Step out to the left side with your left foot. As you do so, turn your hands so your palms are facing each other and bend your elbows, bringing your arms along the sides of your body. Pull your arms back as if you're trying to make your shoulder blades kiss behind you. Return to standing. Time: 15 seconds. Repeat stepping out with the right leg.

▸ Stand with your feet together and hold a dumbbell in each hand. Bend your knees slightly and, with your thighs and knees touching, lean your upper body forward, keeping your back straight. Bend your arms so that they're by your sides with your elbows lifted. Squat down even more with your legs. As you do so, extend your arms straight behind you, squeezing your triceps. Return to the start position. Time: 30 seconds.

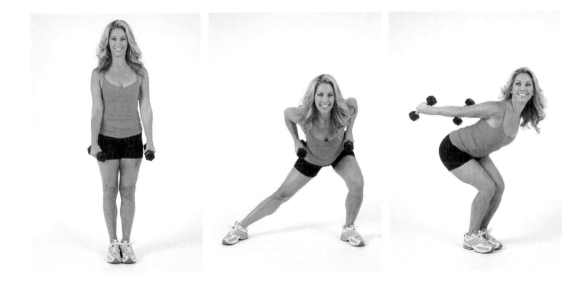

9. Lateral Leaps

You'll get an energy boost and whittle your middle and legs.

▸ Stand with feet shoulder-width apart and your upper body nice and upright. Keep your stomach in and your back flat. Holding a weight in each hand, bend your arms and place your hands in front of your chest.

▸ Step-touch your feet as you squat down low. Really use your legs. As you step-touch, twist your upper body and arms from left to right. Time: 1 minute.

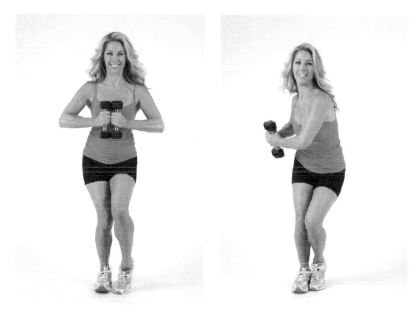

▸ CHALLENGE: Leap from side to side rather than step-touch.

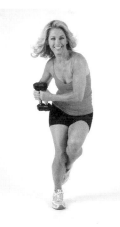

10. Romanian Dead Lift

Target and tone the back of the legs . . . be cellulite free.

▶ Stand facing the right side with your legs shoulder-width apart and your left leg slightly behind your right and just resting on your toe. Pull your abs in and keep your back flat and core strong. Holding a weight in each hand, slide your right arm straight down in front of you with the palm facing your body. Place your left hand on your hip.

▶ With your back flat, slowly lower your upper body in front of you. Then squeeze your buttocks and use the backs of your legs as you pull up and return to standing. Time: 30 seconds. Switch legs and repeat.

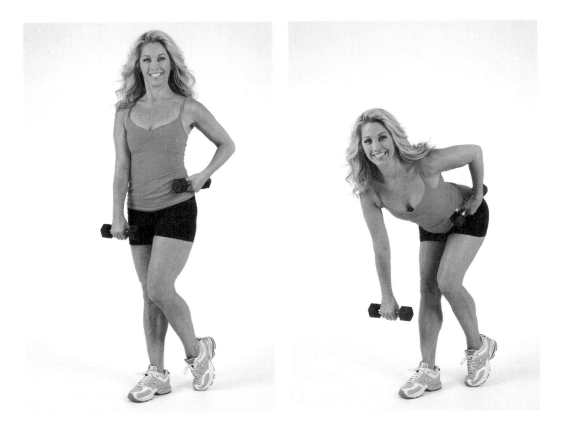

11. Squat Clean and Press

This multitasker targets muscles from head to toe.

▸ Stand with your feet wider than hip-width apart. Hold a dumbbell in your right hand with your right arm extended straight down toward the floor. Place your left hand on your hip. Squat down.

▸ As you stand up, pull your right arm up in a row.

▸ Press the right arm up toward the ceiling. Make sure not to swing your arm. Time: 30 seconds. Switch sides and repeat.

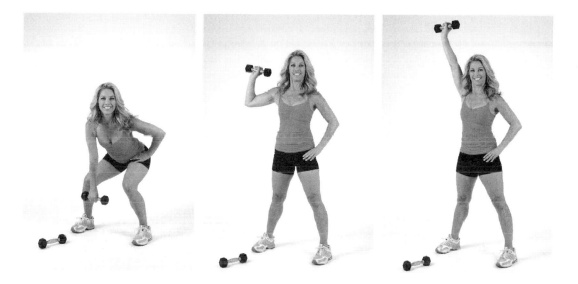

12. Seated Ab Pass-Through
Flat abs are within reach!

▶ Sit on the floor with your legs bent in front of you, heels on the floor, and toes lifted. Hold a dumbbell in your right hand. Keeping your stomach nice and tight, lift your left leg up off the floor and pass the dumbbell from your right hand underneath your bent left leg to your left hand. Use your ab muscles to help you stay upright and lift your leg—it should feel like a crunch. Alternate lifting your legs as you pass the dumbbell from hand to hand. Time: 1 minute.

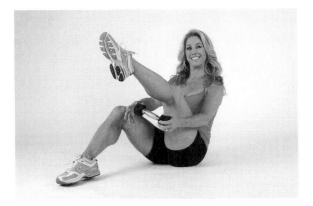

▶ CHALLENGE: Sit on the floor on your knees, holding the weight with both hands. Raising your buttocks off your heels, move the weight from side to side, turning at the waist as if you're paddling a canoe. You should feel this in your obliques (waistline).

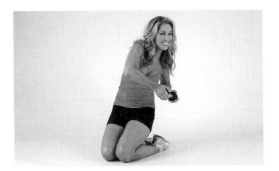

A Dozen Tips from Denise: My Favorite Ways to Relax and De-Stress

Many people eat for reasons that are emotional rather than physical. The key to slimming down is figuring out when you're actually hungry and when you're eating with your emotions. If the latter is true, it's important to know what non-food-related things you can do to soothe yourself. Here, some of the best things to do when you need to chill out and relax.

1. Take a walk. Of course this is great exercise, but sometimes taking a stroll is the ideal way to clear your head and help release brain chemicals called endorphins that can help calm you down. It doesn't have to be a long walk or an intense one. Just put one foot in front of the other to walk stress away.

2. Sniff soothing scents. Several fragrances are known to be calming, such as vanilla and lavender. Try a scented candle or lotion to reap the benefits.

3. Catch a nap. Not getting enough snooze time can leave you feeling anxious and irritable, so sometimes all you need is a quick catnap to take the edge off. Give yourself fifteen minutes to curl up and you'll be amazed how refreshed you feel.

4. Get a rubdown. A massage may seem like an indulgence, but if you can treat yourself, you'll feel amazing afterward. It's relaxing both mentally and physically.

5. Repeat yourself. It's believed that repetitive movements like running a brush through your hair or petting your dog may elicit a relaxation response in your body.

6. Sit quietly. Find a few minutes to sit by yourself and think about nothing. Sometimes you just need to clear your head in order to calm down.

7. Breathe. Often when we're stressed, our breathing becomes very shallow, which just makes us feel worse. Taking a few deep breaths can help slow down your racing heart and make you feel totally refreshed. Plus, bringing oxygen into the body helps energize you, too.

8. Write in a journal. Don't think about what you're writing, don't worry about grammar, and don't focus on making sense. Just write so you can sort out your thoughts and release any tension.

9. Surround yourself with flowers. Research shows that flowers can boost your mood. Perhaps it's their lovely smell or their pretty colors. Either way, putting some blooms in your home can give your mood a lift.

10. Fake it until you make it! When you're feeling bad, get dressed up. Soon your insides will catch up with your outsides.

11. Crack yourself up. Laughter truly is great medicine. Not only does it tone your tummy, but studies show that it can help lower your blood pressure, too!

12. Count your blessings. Everyone goes through tough times, but most of us have so many things to be thankful for. Make a list of ten things you're thankful for and your mood will turn around before you know it.

SATURDAY'S DAILY DOZEN MEAL PLANS

*Sometimes it's not the big temptations
that can ruin a diet, it's the little ones.
You have the power to make good decisions!*

Week One Saturday Daily Dozen Meal Plan

I like today's lunch—a Tuna Salad Salad Wrap—because it's a healthy update of a traditionally high-fat sandwich that's a comfort food for so many of us. I still have wonderful memories of my mom's tuna fish sandwich squished between two slices of white bread. This version is better for you and will leave you feeling satisfied thanks to the fiber in the whole wheat wrap, celery, less mayo, and the protein and good fats in the tuna. Your afternoon snack of almonds and dried fruit helps keep you away from the vending machine when you hit that 4 PM slump. Almonds are rich in heart-healthy fats and protein, and the dried fruit has energizing iron and the antioxidants I keep talking about. Eaten together, this fruit and nut combo reminds me of a delicious cookie without the fat, calories, and guilt! At dinnertime, I've added a sweet potato to the mix because it's full of fiber as well as vitamin C and beta-carotene, nutrients that boost your immune system and give your complexion a healthy glow. Though they're great side dishes for dinner, I also find potatoes to be a good snack, especially when you want a little pick-me-up.

EVERYONE HAS TWELVE MINUTES!

No matter how busy your day gets, don't make it a habit to skip your workouts. This will set a bad precedent of putting exercise—and yourself—last on your list of priorities. Trust me, the benefits of exercise will make a positive difference in so many other areas of your life. Make it number one and you make yourself number one! You are worth it!

BREAKFAST

1 egg + 1 egg white scrambled with ½ cup red, yellow, or orange bell pepper
(1½ protein + ½ veggie)

1 slice whole wheat bread, toasted (1 grain)

Men add: 1 slice whole wheat bread, toasted (1 grain)

½ grapefruit (1 fruit)

Blue Citrus Fruit Treat

½ cup blueberries
½ cup sliced oranges

Chop the oranges and combine in a bowl with the blueberries. Then enjoy!

Tuna Salad Salad Wrap

3 ounces canned tuna (packed in water, drained)
1 teaspoon light mayonnaise
1 teaspoon Dijon mustard
½ cup chopped celery
1 teaspoon lemon juice
½ cup salad mix
1 whole wheat wrap
Pepper, to taste

In a small bowl, combine the tuna, mayo, mustard, celery, lemon juice, and salad mix (I suggest using some of the European salad mix left over from yesterday). Mix and season with pepper. Place the tuna mixture on the wrap, then roll up and enjoy.

MORNING SNACK (MEN ONLY)

Blue Citrus Fruit Treat (1 fruit)

LUNCH

Tuna Salad Salad Wrap
(1 protein + 1 grain +
½ veggie)

1 medium apple (1 fruit)

AFTERNOON SNACK

2 tablespoons almonds
(1 healthy fat)

Men add: 2 tablespoons
almonds (1 healthy fat)

¼ cup dried cranberries
(1 fruit)

DINNER

Simply Delicious Seasoned
Grilled Chicken (*women:*
1 protein; *men:* 1½ protein)

6 stalks steamed asparagus,
with 1 teaspoon olive oil and
fresh lemon juice (1 veggie)

1 medium sweet potato (bake
at 425 degrees F for 30–40
minutes) with butter spray
to taste (1 veggie)

Simply Delicious Seasoned Grilled Chicken

Women: 4 ounces chicken
Men: 5 ounces chicken
1 teaspoon olive oil
Store-bought grill seasoning

Preheat the grill for the chicken. Coat the chicken with olive oil and sprinkle with grill seasoning. Grill for approximately 4 minutes on each side, or until the juices run clear.

NUTRITION INFORMATION FOR THE DAY:

WOMEN	MEN
Calories: 1,180 kcal	*Calories:* 1,480 kcal
Total Fat: 28 g	*Total Fat:* 37 g
Saturated Fat: 5 g	*Saturated Fat:* 7 g
Total Carbohydrate: 156 g	*Total Carbohydrate:* 198 g
Protein: 87 g	*Protein:* 103 g
Sodium: 1,512 mg	*Sodium:* 1,685 mg
Fiber: 25 g	*Fiber:* 32 g

DAILY DOZEN TOTALS FOR THE DAY:

WOMEN	MEN
3½ protein	4 protein
3 veggie	3 veggie
4 fruit	4 fruit
2 grain	3 grain
1 healthy fat	2 healthy fat

Week Two Saturday Daily Dozen Meal Plan

You've been eating healthy foods for almost two weeks, so by now you're probably craving the good-for-you Daily Dozen foods like the fruit medley for today's breakfast. It's a tropical and tasty blend of pineapple, mixed berries, and grapes sprinkled with my favorite topping: flaxseed. These fruits are some of the most colorful—a good indicator that they are loaded with nutrients. Research shows that the deep pigments in fruits and vegetables provide benefits beyond what vitamins and minerals offer. Of course on top of that, they're yummy. I also say that about dinner's Asian Lettuce Wrap, another fabulous meat-free dish that will fill you up—without filling you out. Here, you can sauté any vegetables you like. Some of my favorites are broccoli, snow peas, carrots, and mushrooms, but any produce that you add to the mix will help you on your quest to a slimmer, trimmer you!

You're not only making over your body, you're working to feel great for life!

BREAKFAST
1 cup nonfat cottage cheese (2 protein)
2 tablespoons ground flaxseed, for topping (1 healthy fat)
1 cup fruit medley (pineapple, mixed berries, grapes) (1 fruit)

Garden Salad with Fresh Berries

1½ cups mixed greens
½ cup sliced cucumber
1 cup sliced strawberries
1 teaspoon olive oil
2 teaspoons balsamic vinegar

Place the greens in a bowl and top with cucumbers and strawberries. Drizzle on the olive oil and vinegar and toss well.

MORNING SNACK
1 cup sliced mango (1 fruit)

LUNCH
Garden Salad with Fresh Berries (2 veggie + 1 fruit + 1 healthy fat)
Men add: 4 ounces grilled chicken breast (1 protein)
1 granola bar (make sure it has no more than 200 calories) (1 grain)

AFTERNOON SNACK

1 part-skim mozzarella string
cheese (1 protein)

6 whole wheat crackers
(1 grain)

Men add: 1 kiwi (1 fruit)

DINNER

Asian Lettuce Wrap (2 veggie
+ 1 grain)

Asian Lettuce Wrap

2 cups mixed vegetables
1 tablespoon reduced-sodium soy sauce
1 cup cooked brown rice
2 iceberg lettuce leaves

Sauté the vegetables with the soy sauce in a
nonstick pan. Once they're tender, add the
sautéed vegetables and brown rice to a lettuce leaf. Then roll the leaf to wrap it up.

NUTRITION INFORMATION FOR THE DAY:

WOMEN

Calories: 1,291 kcal

Total Fat: 26 g

Saturated Fat: 7 g

Total Carbohydrate: 215 g

Protein: 60 g

Sodium: 1,078 mg

Fiber: 39 g

MEN

Calories: 1,586 kcal

Total Fat: 31 g

Saturated Fat: 8 g

Total Carbohydrate: 240 g

Protein: 97 g

Sodium: 1,168 mg

Fiber: 45 g

DAILY DOZEN TOTALS FOR THE DAY:

WOMEN

3 protein

4 veggie

3 fruit

3 grain

2 healthy fat

MEN

4 protein

4 veggie

4 fruit

3 grain

2 healthy fat

Week Three Saturday Daily Dozen Meal Plan

Think of healthy food as fuel to power through your busy life!

Today's breakfast is proof positive that you can eat foods that taste indulgent but are actually healthy. My Savory Breakfast, which is lean ham, turkey, or Canadian bacon and cheese on an English muffin, is perfect for a leisurely Saturday morning. Enjoy a vitamin-C-packed grapefruit as your snack—remember, this nutrient can bolster your immune system but also plays a role in collagen production, so it just may ward off wrinkles. Add the almonds and you're getting a wonderful source of vitamin E, magnesium, fiber, and phosphorous, as well as monounsaturated fat, protein, iron, and calcium. Yes, all that in one tiny little almond! For lunch, you'll eat one of my favorite chicken salads. It combines delicious grilled chicken, crisp salad greens, and crunchy walnuts, which are fiber- and protein-packed. For your snack, have a Kashi granola bar. I really like these and all the flavors they come in, but if you don't or can't find them, any granola bar with two hundred calories or less will do. Combine this with the fruit cup and the carbs, protein, and fiber will help you sail through those 4 PM cravings and keep you far away from the vending machine. And

MANAGE MINDLESS EATING

Avoid eating right out of a box or bag—something research shows can cause us to eat 20 percent more. Make sure anything you eat is put on a plate or in a bowl and enjoyed while seated.

HAVE AN *I CAN DO IT* ATTITUDE!

I always look at the bright side of life, but now there's research to show that doing so can help you with your fitness and weight loss goals. A recent study found that people who really believed they would reach their goal of making exercise and eating right a regular part of their lives were more likely to be doing just that one year later!

I just know you're going to love tonight's dinner: Unstuffed Cabbage. This is a family favorite that's so simple to make but absolutely delectable. It combines lean ground turkey, cabbage, and brown rice with yummy spices like garlic, thyme, and pepper.

BREAKFAST
Savory Breakfast (1 grain +
    1 protein)
1 medium banana (1 fruit)

MORNING SNACK
½ grapefruit (1 fruit)
2 tablespoons almonds
    (1 healthy fat)
Men add: 2 tablespoons
    almonds (1 healthy fat)

Savory Breakfast
1 whole-grain English muffin
2 tablespoons shredded light Jarlsberg
    cheese (or any light cheese you have)
1 ounce cooked lean ham, turkey breast,
    or Canadian bacon

Split the English muffin and top each half with cheese. Toast in the oven or a toaster oven until the cheese is melted. Top with your choice of meat.

LUNCH
Grilled Chicken Salad with
    Walnuts (1 protein + 2 veggie + 2 healthy fat)
Men add: 2 tangerines (1 fruit)

AFTERNOON SNACK
1 granola bar (1 grain)
1 cup diced mixed fruit cup (strawberries, grapes, tangerines) (1 fruit)

Grilled Chicken Salad with Walnuts

Women: 3 ounces grilled chicken breast
Men: 4 ounces grilled chicken breast
1½ cups mixed greens
½ cup chopped tomato
2 tablespoons chopped walnuts
2 tablespoons balsamic vinaigrette (no more than 100 calories per 2-tablespoon
   serving)

In a salad bowl, combine the ingredients, drizzle with dressing, and toss.

DINNER

Unstuffed Cabbage (1 protein + 2 veggie + 1 grain)
Men add: 1 cup skim milk (1 protein)

Unstuffed Cabbage

3 ounces ground turkey breast
2 tablespoons chopped onion
1 teaspoon minced garlic
1½ cups chopped cabbage
¼ cup tomato sauce
⅓ cup brown rice, dry
Pinch of thyme
Salt and pepper, to taste
1 cup low-sodium chicken broth

Preheat the oven to 350 degrees Fahrenheit. Spray a small baking dish with cooking spray. Brown the meat in a sauté pan with the onion and garlic; transfer to the baking dish. Add the cabbage, tomato sauce, rice, and thyme. Season with salt and pepper and stir to combine. Pour the broth over the meat mixture. Cover with aluminum foil and bake for 1 hour. Remove the foil and stir. Continue baking, uncovered, for 15 minutes or until the rice is tender.

NUTRITION INFORMATION FOR THE DAY:

WOMEN
Calories: 1,418 kcal
Total Fat: 41 g
Saturated Fat: 6 g
Total Carbohydrate: 192 g
Protein: 85 g
Sodium: 1,895 mg
Fiber: 25 g

MEN
Calories: 1,708 kcal
Total Fat: 49 g
Saturated Fat: 7 g
Total Carbohydrate: 229 g
Protein: 106 g
Sodium: 2,047 mg
Fiber: 30 g

DAILY DOZEN TOTALS FOR THE DAY:

WOMEN
3 protein
4 veggie
3 fruit
3 grain
3 healthy fat

MEN
4 protein
4 veggie
4 fruit
3 grain
4 healthy fat

A BEAUTIFUL VIEW

When you look at beautiful vistas, it causes your brain to release chemicals that can enhance your mood and immune system. Environments can have a positive effect and make you feel better.

A Dozen Tips from Denise:
How to See the Glass—and Your Life—as Half Full

People always comment on my sunny outlook on life. It's something I *choose,* and you can, too. Every single day, I make a decision to embrace what's good about life because I believe that a positive attitude and optimistic outlook can awaken you to so many new possibilities—opportunities that self-doubt and negativity completely miss. The truth is that there are many things in life that we can't control, but your attitude is all up to you. Attitude is everything! Here are twelve tips for looking on the bright side.

1. Take a minute to sit down and make a list of things you like about yourself—for instance, your great smile, your toned arms, and the fact that you're a wonderful friend. Read it every day and add to it regularly.

2. Your mind can only hold one thought at a time. Make it a positive and constructive one. When pessimistic thoughts pop up, imagine a red STOP sign and immediately replace them with thoughts that are more upbeat and productive.

3. When you get out of bed in the morning, tell yourself, "I am worth it!" You really are! Also, write these words on small pieces of paper and keep them where you'll see them often, like above your computer, in your wallet, and on your dresser.

4. Treat yourself to something you really enjoy. A little bit of luxury that reminds you of how special you are. You deserve the best things in life! This doesn't mean you have to spend a lot of money or time, but you'll be amazed how even a small treat like a new lipstick, lotion, a good book, or a talk with a friend can make you feel.

5. A person's greatest emotional need is to feel appreciated. But don't wait for someone else to do it. Instead, appreciate yourself. Appreciate your hard work, strong muscles, and determination to get in shape and lose weight. Respect yourself for improving your body.

6. Instead of thinking of your body as the enemy, think of it as your best friend. You wouldn't constantly criticize or put down your best friend, so don't do the same thing to yourself.

7. Count your blessings; you have many things to be grateful for. It's worth it because research shows that people who experience gratitude do better with tasks that require self-control (like healthy eating and exercise).

8. Replace negative words like *woulda, coulda,* and *shoulda* with positive ones like *I can* and *I will.* Also, challenge your pessimistic thoughts by visualizing yourself doing the unthinkable. It takes baby steps to reach a goal, but you *can* do it and you *will.*

9. Don't dwell on pain and anger from the past. Research shows that people who do so have higher blood pressure, heart rates, and muscle tension. And if your mind is unable to forgive, you hold on to negative energy and your body can become physically stressed. Sure, it can be hard to forgive someone who has really hurt you, but forgiveness improves your health and your life. And *that's* what matters.

10. Try to see the positive or humorous side of everything that happens. You'll be amazed at how that tiny shift in perspective can have an enormous impact on your life.

11. Laugh out loud and do so often. Not only does research show that laughter is good for your immune system and your heart, but it tightens your tummy as well.

12. Assist others who are less fortunate than you are. This helps you appreciate what you have and can change your outlook on life. Walk dogs at a local shelter, volunteer to restore old homes, tutor underprivileged children, or help out at a soup kitchen. The list of ways you can reach out to others is endless; the satisfaction you'll get? Well, that's priceless.

TWELVE REASONS TO BREAK A SWEAT

By now you know that exercise can help you slim down—and hopefully you're seeing this for yourself. But you get so much more from working out than a slimmer waist or smaller size. New studies come out all the time touting all the benefits of breaking a sweat. Use them as motivation to keep up your workout sessions. Because if you do, you'll reap amazing rewards. Read on to find out what they are.

1. Working out helps you reawaken thousands of muscle cells so you'll have more energy and vitality.

2. Exercise can lift your spirits because it releases brain chemicals called endorphins. These naturally enhance your mood, which is why you always feel better after a workout than you did when you started.

3. Breaking a sweat is an ideal way to relieve tension and de-stress.

4. Food tastes better, and you'll know that you've earned it.

5. Exercise helps you build more muscle, which boosts your metabolism.

6. Exercise will help your clothes fit better.

7. Moving around helps clear your head and may make you feel more creative. I know that I get some of my best ideas while working out.

8. Working out enhances circulation, giving your complexion a youthful, rosy glow.

9. Exercise helps reduce your risk of an array of diseases from diabetes to cancer to heart disease. There's no better preventive medicine than good old-fashioned exercise.

10. You'll sweat your way to a younger-looking body.

11. Your posture will improve so you'll stand taller.

12. Working out improves your health, so you'll live longer to enjoy life with your family and your friends. How's that for motivation?

My Daily Dozen Saturday Checklist

	WEEK ONE	WEEK TWO	WEEK THREE
I ate my Daily Dozen Foods			
VEGGIE			
VEGGIE			
VEGGIE			
FRUIT			
FRUIT			
FRUIT			
PROTEIN			
PROTEIN			
PROTEIN			
HEALTHY GRAIN			
HEALTHY GRAIN			
HEALTHY FAT			
EIGHT 8-OUNCE GLASSES OF WATER			
I did my Daily Dozen exercises			
I did some of my weekly twelve miles of cardio (write how many miles)			
I did some fidget-cisers today (write how many)			

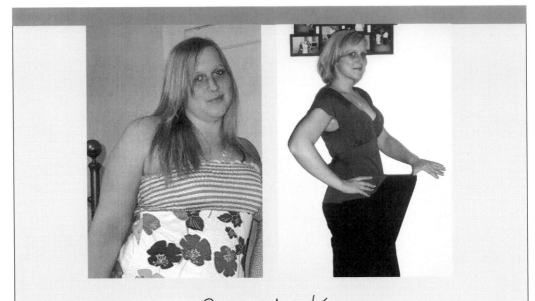

Cassandra King,
24, marketing associate, Massillon, Ohio
POUNDS LOST: 80

When I was three, I had a tumor removed from my thoracic cavity, which resulted in diminished lung capacity. As a child and adolescent, I used this medical condition as an excuse to get out of running laps, racing other kids, enrolling in sports, or doing any other vigorous exercise. This combined with the fact that my overweight family indulged more in comfort food than healthy food meant that I gained weight. My mother died when I was only twenty and I fell into a severe depression, indulging in comfort foods to avoid my true feelings, friends, and family. I knew the pounds were stacking up, but I tried to ignore it. I also started having agonizing knee pain due to deteriorating cartilage. An orthopedic surgeon said that if I lost weight, every pound lost would alleviate seven pounds of pressure from my knees and I might be able to avoid surgery and arthritis. On top of the severe depression, weight gain, and knee problems, I discovered a family history of diabetes, high blood pressure, high cholesterol, Alzheimer's, cancer, heart attacks, and congestive heart failure.

"I decided that enough was enough! I didn't want to die at a young age from conditions that were preventable. I decided to become a happier, healthier me because, like Denise says, 'I'm worth it!' I had never tried to diet, exercise, or lose weight before, but this was *not* a diet. This was a promise to myself to change my life for the better, be healthier, and live longer! I enrolled in a wellness program at work, watched what I ate, and took a class at the gym and exercised with Denise's DVDs. I loved the challenge and uplifting positivity of Denise's workouts. I started seeing results in the first few weeks! My clothes were a little looser, and I saw a major difference in my face, waistline, and thighs. I love all of my Denise Austin workouts, but *The Daily Dozen* is one of my absolute favorites. The simple twelve-minute workouts offer an assortment of challenges, from kickboxing to toning to aerobics to the relaxing yoga stretch. I enjoy the workouts so much that I'll do the whole DVD at once since I've progressed to working out for at least an hour every day. I also enjoyed learning about the twelve foods to eat every day. I've lost a total of eighty pounds, ten pant sizes, going from a size eighteen to an eight! My BMI is now 23.5, which is well within the healthy weight range for my height. I also recently donated twelve inches of my hair to Locks of Love. I grew my hair throughout my weight loss and cut it when I reached my goal of seventy pounds. I'm extremely proud to say that with the help of Denise Austin, I've been able to beat depression, truly commit to being fit, and find a healthier, happier mol"

*I'm confident that if you haven't already seen
the beautiful things that are happening to your body
and your mind, you will very soon!*

Sunday

Today is soothing Sunday, and after all your efforts this week, you deserve it! Take a moment and pat yourself on the back for following this plan so far. It might seem as if it was a long first week (or two), but look at all that you've accomplished. First, you made the important decision to jump-start your life, and you *did* it! Yes! Then you chose to eat a wholesome diet of good-for-you foods in the place of unhealthy items that used to be lurking in your pantry—a vital step toward better health. Plus, you got moving. You did some cardio, some strength training, and some stretching. Appreciate yourself and the effort you're making to change your life and get healthy and fit. I believe that the best way to predict your future is to create it and to make it happen. And that's exactly what

Don't put off exercise until tomorrow when you can exercise today. Get moving now!

WEIGHT LOSS IS MORE THAN SKIN-DEEP

As you work on shaping up and becoming a healthier person, keep in mind that there is more to becoming healthy than changing your appearance. Just as you can gauge your weight loss by stepping on a scale regularly, you can, and should, measure your progress another way—by taking stock of how you feel! Is your energy level increasing? Are you sleeping better? These things are just as important as your size—if not more so, because they're signs of good health. Be proud of yourself for how far you've come!

GO BACK TO GRADE SCHOOL

Revisit your elementary school days and start jumping rope. This is an efficient but challenging calorie-burning workout. It's also perfect for people who can't exercise outdoors due to bad weather or safety concerns. Also, doing a few minutes of jumping here or there can give you an energy boost during the day. If you have trouble coordinating your arms with your feet, start by jumping without the rope, then add it in later. For variety, try doing jumping jack jumps, small jumps, large jumps, and jogging with the rope. It may take a little practice, but you'll feel like a kid again.

you've been doing on the Daily Dozen Plan so far. Give yourself a round of applause and know that there are many more great things in store.

Now, in order to treat your body right after all this hard work, today's Daily Dozen is a yoga stretch routine that soothes and relaxes your muscles from head to toe. I love yoga and usually do it on weekends, too. Yoga, which originated in India, is an ancient philosophy involving the unity of mind, body, and spirit. It incorporates an approach to achieving enlightenment through specific breathing exercises, meditation, and physical postures called asanas, also known as yoga poses. I've included several asanas in today's Daily Dozen because they help strengthen your muscles, release tension, reduce soreness, and rejuvenate your body. The stretching that follows helps elongate your muscles so they look lean and strong, not bulky. Stretching is also important because it helps improve your flexibility—and being flexible is a critical part of preventing injuries. For example, tight hamstrings can tug on your lower back muscles and cause the back pain that so many people experience daily, and tight quadriceps can cause knee pain. My yoga routine will help you improve your balance, which is the foundation of keeping you young! Additionally, stretching increases circulation, and boosting blood

GET YOUR GROOVE ON

Not in the mood for a walk or a run? Well, you can still get a heart-pumping workout by turning on your favorite high-energy music and boogying. You can't beat a fun dance workout, so shake, twist, and kick your body slim. As long as you get your heart rate up, you're burning calories.

FINDING THE PERFECT GYM

If you've never belonged to a gym or have never even worked out at one, the prospect of signing up for a membership can be scary! *Which one is for me? When should I go? What do I do when I get there?* Believe me, you're not alone. It can be a bit overwhelming at first, but like everything in life, all it takes is practice and you'll be an old pro in no time! If you're considering a gym membership, think about the gym's location (you'll go more if it's close to work or home), hours (make sure it's open at times you need to go), offerings (check to see if it has the machines and classes you want), and staff members (are they friendly and certified through a recognized fitness organization?).

flow throughout your body helps it heal. But equally important to what yoga does for you physically is what it does for you spiritually. It centers you and calms you. It not only rejuvenates your muscles, but rejuvenates your mind.

The following twelve moves are simple to do—I promise, no crazy pretzel poses. As a whole, these moves target your body from head to toe. But you can also do a few of these stretches each day when you get up in the morning, as a break from sitting for long periods of time, before bed at night to target what ails you, or simply to keep your muscles supple. You'll see that these moves stretch more than one area at a time, and that tiny tweaks in positioning stretch one muscle in a different way or target a new one. This means that just as form is important when you're doing strength or cardio workouts, it's also important when you're doing yoga stretches. Trust me, once you try it, you'll be glad you added yoga, with all its benefits, to your workouts!

Though I give you a suggested amount of time to hold each of the stretches below, note that the longer you hold one, the more your muscles will relax. If you're a beginner and have trouble with balance in some of the poses, hold on to something sturdy like a chair. Also, if you experience tightness, you can encourage your muscles to relax through breathing. Bringing oxygen into the body is very cleansing and energizing and will renew your strength and inspiration. It works the same way as those deep cleansing breaths that help in childbirth! So fill up your lungs and get ready to soothe and pamper your body from head to toe. Why? Because you and your muscles have earned it. You are worth it!

SUNDAY'S YOGA STRETCH WORKOUT

There is nothing more rewarding than taking good care of yourself!

1. Warm Up

It's very important to move your spine in all directions: lateral moves (sideways), extension of the spine (bending slightly backward), flexion (bending forward), and rotation of the spine (twist). Do these stretches in the following sequence.

▶ HALF-MOON: Stand with your feet together. Lift your arms out to the sides and then up toward the ceiling. Lean your body to the right side, then lean to the left and repeat. This moves your spine laterally. Time: 10 seconds on each side.

▶ SPINE STRETCHES: Stand with your feet together. Lift your arms straight up toward the ceiling and lean back slightly. These stretches are for extension and flexion. Time: 20 seconds.

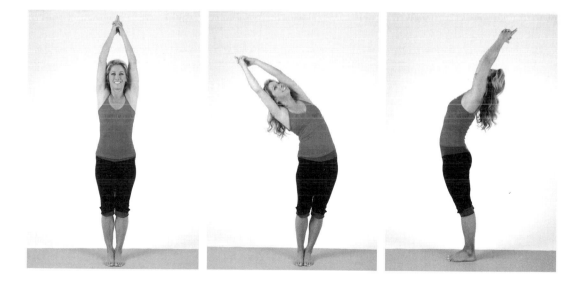

▸ Squat down so your body is like a tiny ball. Straighten your legs as your upper body hangs over them with your hands on your calves or under your heels. Time: 20 seconds.

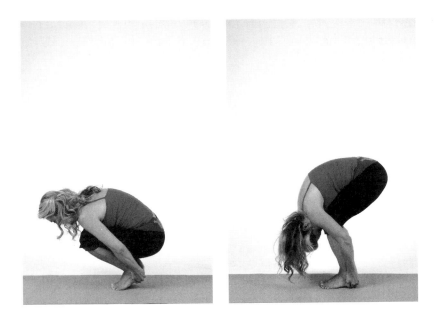

▸ CHALLENGE: Straighten your legs completely as you hang over them.

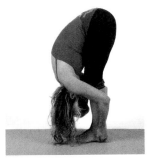

2. Rotation Spine Stretch

Give your legs and back a soothing stretch.

▶ Stand with your legs two to three feet apart, toes facing forward. Abs strong, bend over at the waist and, keeping your back flat, twist your upper body to the left. Place your right hand on the floor and extend the left hand up toward the ceiling. Time: 30 seconds. Switch sides and repeat.

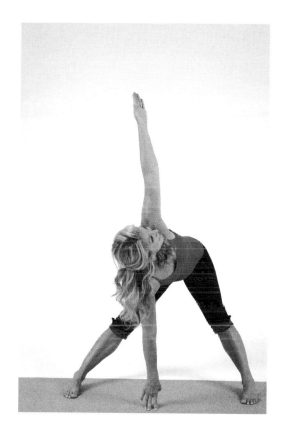

3. Standing Quad Stretch

*This is great for the front of your thighs and hip flexors
that get very tight from sitting too much.*

▶ Stand with your feet shoulder-width apart. Grasp your left foot with your left hand. Bend your leg behind you, bringing the foot toward your buttocks. Extend your right arm toward the ceiling to help you balance. Push your hips slightly forward so you feel an extra stretch in the front of the thigh. If you need help with balance, use a wall or sturdy chair. Time: 30 seconds. Switch sides and repeat.

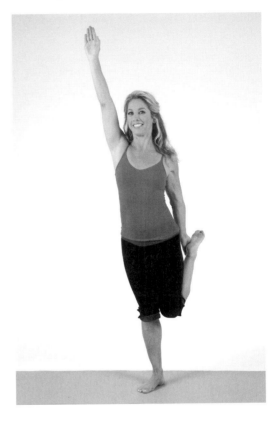

▶ CHALLENGE: Lean your body forward and lift the leg behind you. Extend the opposite arm in front of you.

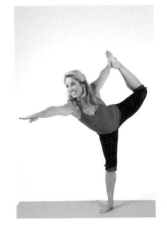

4. Hip and Thigh Stretch
This is my favorite stretch of all time!

▶ Stand with your feet hip-width apart, then bend the left knee and place your right ankle on your left thigh. Extend your arms up and out to the sides on a diagonal. Squat down to feel an even deeper stretch. To help with balance, hold on to a sturdy chair or use the wall. Time: 30 seconds. Switch legs and repeat.

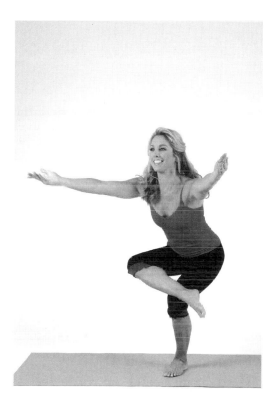

5. Warrior

*This strengthens your back and legs and
gives you an awesome inner-thigh stretch.*

▸ Stand with your feet shoulder-width apart.
With your right foot, step out to the right side
about three feet. Extend your arms out to the
sides at shoulder height; your feet should be directly under your fingertips. Turn your right foot
out at a forty-five-degree angle. Keeping your left
leg straight, bend your right leg so it is directly in
line with your ankle, forming a ninety-degree
angle, and lower yourself in a lunge position.
Time: 15 seconds.

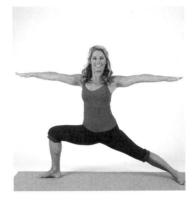

▸ REVERSE WARRIOR: Hold the above Warrior pose
and raise your right arm up as you slide your left
hand along the back of your left leg, stopping
where it's comfortable for you. Lean back slightly
and look up to your right hand. Let your lower
body sink into the pose as your upper body lifts
up toward the ceiling. Time: 15 seconds.

▸ Switch legs and repeat both stretches.

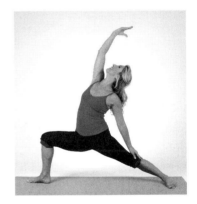

▸ CHALLENGE: Facing forward, place your right hand
near your right toes and extend your left arm up
toward the ceiling. Look up toward your left arm.

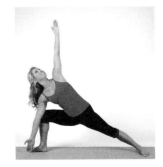

6. Back Stretch/Camel

This strengthens your thighs and improves back mobility.

▸ Kneel on the floor but sit all the way up so your body forms a right angle. Extend your arms straight in front of you at shoulder height and lean back. Time: 15 seconds. Then release and relax for 5 seconds. Repeat twice.

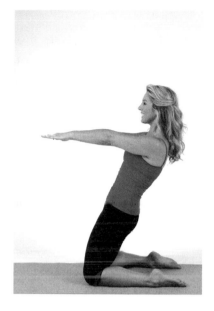

▸ CHALLENGE: Lean all the way back into a back bend with your hands on your heels and your head looking up at the ceiling.

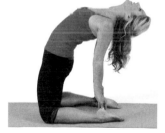

7. Abs and Back Stretch
Say good-bye to back pain!

▸ Kneel on the floor with your buttocks resting on your heels and arms extended up toward the ceiling.

▸ As you bend forward at the waist, tighten your abs and use your core muscles the whole way down until your hands reach the floor. Extend your arms straight above your head with palms facing down. Push down on the floor with your arms so that you feel the stretch in the sides of the arms and upper back. This is a variation of yoga's Downward Dog called the Puppy. Time: 30 seconds. Then come back up and repeat. As you come back up, use your abs, trying to keep your back as straight as possible.

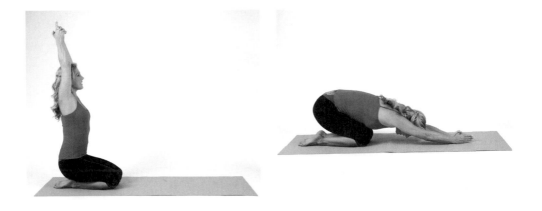

8. Shoulder and Triceps Stretch

This yoga pose, called Needle, really stretches the middle of the back and relieves tension between the shoulder blades.

▸ From the Puppy position, reach your left arm underneath your right armpit and extend the arm flat on the floor with the palm facing upward as you place your left shoulder on the floor. Time: 15 seconds. Switch arms and repeat.

▸ Lie with your upper body and head down on the mat. Extend your left arm straight with the palm down. Bend your right elbow, bringing the palm toward your right shoulder. Time: 15 seconds. Switch arms and repeat.

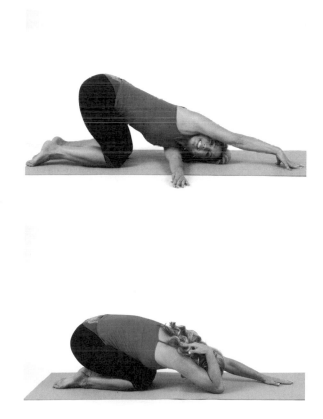

9. Chest and Back Stretch

This strengthens the muscles that line your spine to keep it young and supple while also improving your posture.

▸ Lie on the floor on your stomach with your legs extended behind you and arms bent, your palms on the floor under your shoulders. Lift your upper body off the floor slightly. Time: 1 minute.

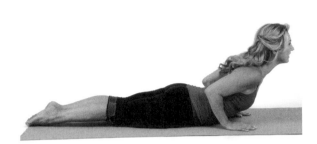

▸ CHALLENGE: Straighten your arms and press your upper body back and off the floor.

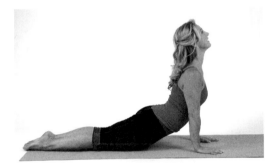

10. Downward Dog
You can't get a better full-body stretch than this one.

▶ From the chest and back stretch position, lift your hips up off the floor and straighten your arms. Stretch your heels back toward the floor. Keep your head in line with your arms. Time: 30 seconds. Take a few seconds to relax and repeat.

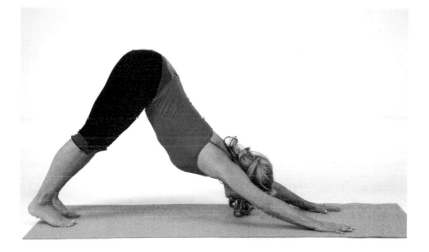

11. Pigeon

I love the way this opens the hips and releases tension.

▸ Sit with your right leg bent in front of you so your calf is parallel to your torso, and your left leg extended straight behind you. Keep your chest lifted and your hands on the floor on either side of your leg.

▸ Lean forward over your front leg. Time: 30 seconds. Switch legs and repeat.

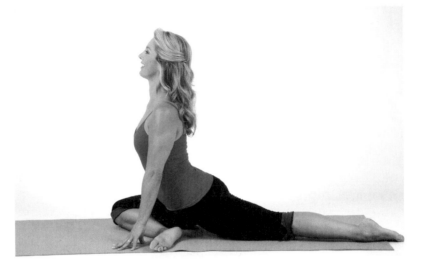

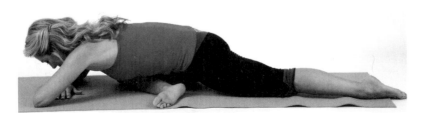

12. Neck, Chest, and Shoulders

These are three of my favorite stretches! They just feel so good!

▶ NECK: Sit up tall with your legs crossed in front of you. Place your right hand on the left side of your head above your left ear and gently pull your head to the right side. Feel lengthening all through the left side of your neck. Time: 10 seconds. Switch sides and repeat.

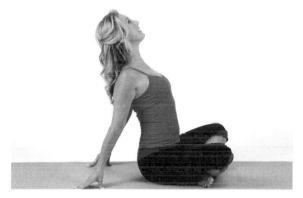

▶ CHEST: From the same seated position, place your hands on the floor behind you and lean back. Lift your chest up toward the ceiling. Time: 20 seconds.

▶ SHOULDERS: From the same seated position, bring your right arm across your chest. Hold your elbow with your left hand. Time: 10 seconds. Repeat on the other side.

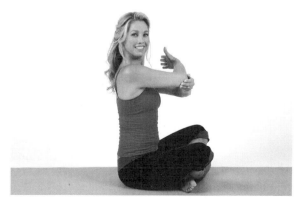

A Dozen Tips from Denise:
Healthy Rewards for Your Hard Work

Sometimes staying motivated requires a little incentive. There's nothing wrong with that! The next time you get through a really tough workout, beat your previous running time, or follow your healthy-eating plan flawlessly for a straight week, give yourself a well-deserved pat on the back—do something special that's all about you! Here, some great ideas—because you'll find that a little treat goes a long way!

1. Splurge on professional pampering. Get a fabulous new haircut, a mani-pedi, a facial, or a massage. Treating your body will feel so good.

2. Pamper yourself at home—there's no need to go to an expensive spa! Ask your mother or a friend to let the kids stay overnight, and spend an evening soaking in a tub filled with lavender-scented essential oil.

3. If you're close to your ideal weight, shop for some new clothes to fit your incredibly shrinking body!

4. Reward your hard work each month by picking up a new fitness accessory—a medicine ball, pedometer, or my *Yoga Body Burn* DVD.

5. Shop for a cute new piece of fitness wear to flatter your slimming figure.

6. Visit a home store and buy yourself a kitchen tool to help you prepare all those good-for-you meals.

7. Seek out a beautiful spot—like a park, a spot with sweeping vistas, a beach, a forest, or any place with more light—and get back to nature.

8. Slip out of your house or office for half an hour and head to your favorite coffee bar. Spend some time with a magazine or novel that you've been dying to finish and a low-fat latte.

9. Treat yourself to a new low-fat cookbook or cooking magazine. It's always exciting to discover new ways to eat right.

10. Make today's cardio workout a family affair by taking a brisk walk with your husband, playing tag with your kids, or going bike riding with your best friend.

11. Try something new. Borrow a new fitness DVD from the library or tag along with a friend to her favorite fitness class.

12. Write yourself a letter saying how proud you are of your accomplishments and all the benefits you've reaped from this hard work. Keep this handy for days when your motivation lags. Update it regularly.

*From your own efforts, you will make a difference
and you will feel good about yourself!*

Week One Sunday Daily Dozen Meal Plan

If Sundays used to mean indulgent brunches—read *high-fat* and *high-calorie*—
don't worry. Today's meals are rich and satisfying and good for you, too. Topping
healthy waffles with fresh kiwi gives them a tangy
flavor and makes them feel a little bit special. The
hearty black bean soup to accompany your lunch lets
you reap the endless benefits of beans. Research says
beans may help your heart by regulating your blood
pressure, decreasing levels of unhealthy hormones, and sopping up cholesterol—
your bad cholesterol goes down and your good cholesterol goes up.

**All you can ask of yourself is
that you try your very best!**

BREAKFAST
2 whole-grain frozen waffles (toasted) (2 grain)
1 kiwi, topping (1 fruit)

LUNCH
Roasted Turkey Roll-Ups with Sliced Avocado (1 protein + 1 healthy fat)
2 cups low-sodium Amy's Organic Black Bean Vegetable Soup (2 veggie +
   1 protein)
1 medium apple (1 fruit)

Roasted Turkey Roll-Ups with Sliced Avocado

1 teaspoon Dijon mustard (spicy is a favorite of mine)
3 ounces roasted turkey breast
¼ avocado, sliced

Spread the mustard on the individual slices of turkey breast, place sliced avocado in
the turkey, roll up, and enjoy!

AFTERNOON SNACK

½ grapefruit (1 fruit)

Men add: ½ grapefruit and 1 tablespoon almonds (1 fruit + 1 healthy fat)

DINNER

Marinated Flank Steak Kebabs and Baked Potato (1 protein + 3 veggie)

Marinated Flank Steak Kebabs and Baked Potato

1 medium Idaho potato
4 ounces broiled flank steak
1 red, yellow, or orange bell pepper
1 cup white button mushrooms
1 tablespoon olive oil
1 tablespoon balsamic vinegar
1 fresh rosemary sprig
Salt and pepper, to taste
Butter spray (optional)

Preheat the oven to 425 degrees Fahrenheit. Clean the skin of the potato, poke a few holes in it with a fork, and place it in the oven for approximately 30 to 40 minutes, or until it can be pierced with a sharp knife. Cut the flank steak into 1-inch cubes. Wash and cut all the vegetables into approximate 1-inch pieces. Mix the olive oil, balsamic vinegar, rosemary, salt, and pepper in a separate bowl. Skewer the steak cubes and vegetables, alternating steak, pepper, and mushroom until the skewers are full. Brush marinade over the skewers and grill until the steak is cooked all the way through. If desired, spritz the potato with butter spray, and add salt and pepper to taste.

YOU ARE WHAT YOU EAT!

And that includes your skin. Experts say that certain highly processed foods and those with refined sugars may be a complexion problem for those who are acne-prone. Keep your skin glowing and gorgeous by eating whole grains, lean sources of protein, and lots of vitamin-rich produce, as well as at least eight 8-ounce glasses of water a day.

NUTRITION INFORMATION FOR THE DAY:

WOMEN	MEN
Calories: 1,229 kcal	*Calories:* 1,446 kcal
Total Fat: 24 g	*Total Fat:* 38 g
Saturated Fat: 7 g	*Saturated Fat:* 7 g
Total Carbohydrate: 215 g	*Total Carbohydrate:* 228 g
Protein: 64 g	*Protein:* 71 g
Sodium: 1,096 mg	*Sodium:* 1,109 mg
Fiber: 51 g	*Fiber:* 55 g

DAILY DOZEN TOTALS FOR THE DAY:

WOMEN	MEN
3 protein	3 protein
5 veggie	5 veggie
3 fruit	4 fruit
2 grain	2 grain
1 healthy fat	2 healthy fat

Week Two Sunday Daily Dozen Meal Plan

The road to success has many tempting parking places and rest stops. Just keep going! That's not too hard when you've got a menu that's filled with delicious foods. Today's certainly is. The Breakfast Burrito is a spicy way to start the day, and you're getting the benefits of protein, carbs, and even antioxidants like lycopene from the salsa. For lunch, a protein-topped salad helps you make it through the afternoon without your stomach growling. And for dinner you've got the very light and low-cal halibut along with quinoa, a grain that boasts more protein than most others. In fact, it's considered a complete protein because it has all the essential amino acids.

Nothing feels better than the time after a workout. It's a great feeling of self-accomplishment. You overcame procrastination.

BREAKFAST
Breakfast Burrito (*women:*
    1½ protein + 1 grain; *men:*
    2 protein + 1 grain)
1 cup strawberries (1 fruit)
Men add: 1 cup skim milk
    (1 protein)

MORNING SNACK
1 medium apple (1 fruit)
1 tablespoon natural peanut
    butter (1 healthy fat)

LUNCH
Salad with Turkey & Feta
    (2½ veggie + 1 protein +
    2 healthy fat)
1 medium orange (1 fruit)

AFTERNOON SNACK
½ cup grapes (½ fruit)
Men add: 1 granola bar
    (no more than 200 calories)
    (1 grain)

Breakfast Burrito

1 sprouted grain tortilla
1 egg plus 1 egg white, scrambled
Men add: 1 egg, scrambled
1 tablespoon salsa

Warm the tortilla in microwave for 30 seconds. Add cooked eggs to the tortilla, top with salsa, and roll up.

Salad with Turkey & Feta

2 cups baby spinach
½ cup chopped cucumber
2 ounces roasted turkey breast
2 tablespoons crumbled low-fat feta cheese
2 teaspoons extra virgin olive oil
2 teaspoons balsamic vinegar

In a large bowl, combine the spinach, cucumber, turkey, and feta. Drizzle with oil and vinegar.

CELEBRATE SUCCESS

Life is too short not to celebrate the many wonderful reasons we have to be happy! We're all too quick to put ourselves down for "cheating" on our diets or skipping a night at the gym, but we forget about celebrating the many positives in our lives, as well as the small victories we achieve daily. Congratulating yourself along your weight loss journey—every time you complete a difficult workout, lose a pound, or stay strong and stick to your diet during a tempting situation—will help keep you motivated!

DINNER

Baked Halibut with Quinoa (*women:* 1 protein + 1 veggie; *men:* 1½ protein + 1 veggie)

Baked Halibut with Quinoa

1 cup quinoa
2 cups chicken broth
Women: 4 ounces halibut
Men: 5 ounces halibut
1 teaspoon Very Very Teriyaki sauce
1 teaspoon toasted sesame oil
½ tablespoon olive oil
1 cup pea pods
1 teaspoon black sesame seeds

Preheat the oven to 350 degrees Fahrenheit. Rinse the quinoa. Pour the chicken broth into a medium saucepan and bring to a boil. Once it's boiling, add the rinsed quinoa, reduce to a simmer, and cook for approximately 20 minutes, or until all the liquid is absorbed. Meanwhile, spray a black iron skillet with nonstick spray. Add the halibut, drizzle with teriyaki sauce, and place the skillet in the preheated oven. Bake for 20 minutes. While it bakes, add the sesame oil and olive oil to a sauté pan and turn the heat to medium. Add the pea pods and toss to coat. Add the black sesame seeds and cook until the pea pods are tender, but still crisp when broken. Serve the halibut on top of the quinoa.

NUTRITION INFORMATION FOR THE DAY:

WOMEN	MEN
Calories: 1,257 kcal	*Calories:* 1,596 kcal
Total Fat: 39 g	*Total Fat:* 49 g
Saturated Fat: 10 g	*Saturated Fat:* 13 g
Total Carbohydrate: 146 g	*Total Carbohydrate:* 187 g
Protein: 87 g	*Protein:* 106 g
Sodium: 1,495 mg	*Sodium:* 1,712 mg
Fiber: 28 g	*Fiber:* 30 g

DAILY DOZEN TOTALS FOR THE DAY:

WOMEN	MEN
3½ protein	5½ protein
3½ veggie	3½ veggie
3½ fruit	3½ fruit
3 grain	3 grain
3 healthy fat	3 healthy fat

Week Three Sunday Daily Dozen Meal Plan

Your great food choices today are your rewards tomorrow. Plan ahead!

By now you know what a powerhouse oatmeal is, but did you know there are endless numbers of ways to prepare it? Today you'll sprinkle on cinnamon and raisins, though a quarter cup of any dried fruit—like cranberries, sliced prunes, or chopped dates—will do. The taste of this morning's fruit medley snack—which contains melon, mango, pineapple, and berries—will make you feel as if you're on a tropical getaway while energizing you at the same time with all its nutrients. Add protein and calcium-rich yogurt and you'll be sweetly satisfied all morning long. The Chicken & Pepper Flatbread for lunch is so easy to make and yet it's also extremely satisfying. Something about that gooey cheese just really hits the spot! And I also love the Citrus Marinated Chicken Kebabs for dinner. They're so juicy and have a unique flavor thanks to the honey, pineapple, and curry powder combination. The pineapple adds a sweet taste and is loaded with vitamins B_1, B_6,

ENJOY THE RIDE!

One of my favorite sayings is "The joy is truly in the journey." Learning about yourself and taking pride in your small accomplishments along the way is all part of the experience. Sure, there are tough times, but it's all part of the effort to change your life for the better. I encourage you to soak up as much of the experience as you can and to include the important people in your life in your journey as well.

and C as well as fiber, while the curry powder contains compounds believed to have cancer-fighting benefits. The onions also offer an array of nutrients including chromium, folate, potassium, and phosphorus and are believed to stave off an array of diseases, too. But that's not the only reason that I often make enough of this chicken dish so that we have leftovers. It's because it's so delicious that it leaves my family asking for more!

BREAKFAST

1 cup cooked oatmeal (prepared with water) (1 grain)

¼ cup raisins, for topping (1 fruit)

1 teaspoon cinnamon, for topping

Men add: ½ cup oatmeal (½ grain)

MORNING SNACK

1 cup fruit medley (melon, pineapple, mango, berries, etc.) (1 fruit)

1 cup nonfat vanilla yogurt (1 protein)

LUNCH

Chicken & Pepper Flatbread (1 grain + 2 protein + ½ veggie)

1 pear (1 fruit)

Chicken & Pepper Flatbread

1 whole wheat pita or Flatout bread
3 ounces diced grilled chicken breast
½ cup sliced bell pepper (any color)
¼ cup shredded part-skim mozzarella cheese
½ teaspoon dried oregano

Preheat the oven to 375 degrees Fahrenheit. Place the pita on a baking sheet lined with aluminum foil. Top with the chicken, pepper, and cheese. Sprinkle with oregano and bake until the cheese is melted and bubbly.

AFTERNOON SNACK

1 sliced bell pepper (1 veggie)

2 tablespoons almonds (1 healthy fat)

Men add: 2 tablespoons almonds (1 healthy fat)

DINNER

Citrus Marinated Chicken Kebabs (1 protein + ½ fruit + 1½ veggie)

1 medium baked potato (1 veggie)

Citrus Marinated Chicken Kebabs

½ small can frozen orange juice concentrate, thawed

2 tablespoons honey

1 tablespoon curry powder

½ cup low-fat Italian salad dressing

¼ cup pickled jalapeño peppers, including 1 tablespoon juice

4 ounces boneless, skinless chicken breast, cut into 1-inch cubes

½ cup 1-inch-diced pineapple

½ cup 1-inch-diced red onion

In a large resealable bag, add the orange juice concentrate, honey, curry, dressing, and peppers. Add the chicken to the bag, seal, and refrigerate for at least 30 minutes. Preheat the grill or a grill pan to medium-high. Place the marinated chicken, pineapple, and onion on skewers and grill for 3 to 4 minutes per side until the chicken is cooked through.

NUTRITION INFORMATION FOR THE DAY:

WOMEN	MEN
Calories: 1,392 kcal	*Calories:* 1,709 kcal
Total Fat: 37 g	*Total Fat:* 45 g
Saturated Fat: 10 g	*Saturated Fat:* 11 g
Total Carbohydrate: 185 g	*Total Carbohydrate:* 233 g
Protein: 88 g	*Protein:* 103 g
Sodium: 583 mg	*Sodium:* 741 mg
Fiber: 30 g	*Fiber:* 34 g

DAILY DOZEN TOTALS FOR THE DAY:

WOMEN	MEN
4 protein	4 protein
4 veggie	4 veggie
3½ fruit	3½ fruit
2 grain	2½ grain
1 healthy fat	2 healthy fat

A Dozen Tips from Denise:
How to Survive Dinner Out When You're on a Diet

Eating at a friend's house is a special treat, so it's not one that you have to give up even when you're trying to slim down. You just need to follow some simple strategies and you're good to go! With some simple preparation and a bit of discipline, dinner at a friend's can be an enjoyable—and diet-friendly—experience! Here are a few ideas on how to strike a balance. You can do it!

1. Pick and choose. When dinner is served, focus on veggie dishes, salads, and meats. Politely pass on anything that's smothered in sauces, cream, or mayo. If you *do* decide to indulge in a rich entrée or a dessert, stick with a single, sensible portion.

2. Bring your own dish. If dinner is potluck, bring a nutritious, diet-friendly option such as a healthy vegetable dish, crudités platter, or fruit salad. This way you'll have something "safe" to eat, and you'll be sharing the gift of health!

3. Watch your hands. If there are munchies within your reach, be sure to have only a single small portion instead of repeatedly reaching for the bowl. Hold a glass of water or carry a clutch purse with one hand so it's harder to pig out.

4. Be careful with the cocktails. Alcoholic drinks can be loaded with calories and lower your inhibitions so you eat more. Have a glass of wine or a white wine spritzer—half wine, half seltzer—instead of a sugary cocktail.

5. Inform your friend. Sometimes we feel pressured to eat because we think friends will be insulted if we don't. Before the dinner party, tell your host not to feel that way when you don't try everything or ask for seconds. Let her know that you're trying to slim down and not all her yummy dishes are on your menu.

6. Or keep quiet. Whether they do it consciously or not, some friends and relatives sabotage our best intentions to live a healthy life. And pressure from family and friends can actually work against you staying motivated and slim. If your host is that type, then don't fill her in on your new way of life. Instead think of a few things you can say, such as that you had a big or late lunch, when she pushes a fattening food on you. You can also politely take a serving and leave it on your plate. Just because it's there doesn't mean you have to eat it.

7. Enjoy the company. The reason we gather with friends is to share their company and conversation, and in our go-go-go world spending time with loved ones is rare. Instead of focusing on the food, pay extra attention to those around you. You won't overindulge, *and* you'll connect with others in a meaningful way.

8. Look before you eat. If the dinner is a buffet, survey the whole spread before you choose what you'll eat. Also, use a small plate so you don't overdo it.

9. Offer your assistance. Helping a friend prepare, serve, and do other things at the dinner may keep you too busy to munch mindlessly. Plus, you'll get a bit of exercise getting up and down or going back and forth to the kitchen.

10. Don't go hungry. Some people starve themselves all day so they can eat what they want at a dinner party or special occasion. The problem? You'll be so hungry when you arrive at your friend's that you're likely to make poor food choices and leave with an aching tummy and loads of regret. Stick with healthy meals during the day and eat a filling snack right before you go.

11. Stay focused on *your* goals. When others around us are pigging out, it's all too easy to throw in the towel and follow their lead. A study done at Vanderbilt University in Nashville found that, on average, women took in 696 calories when they ate with others compared with 476 calories when they dined alone. But that doesn't mean you should shun social meals. Just remember that your goals are different from your friend's. Just because a girlfriend is reaching for seconds—or thirds—doesn't mean that you have to.

12. Think before you eat. Before diving into that decadent dessert, imagine how you'll feel if you step on the scale and it's gone up or hasn't budged, or if your clothes are snug. Often the momentary pleasure is not worth the guilt you'll feel later.

TWELVE KITCHEN TIME SAVERS

It happens all the time. You got caught at work and you're rushing to get dinner on the table. But restaurant meals are expensive and you don't have control over what's in them—bad news when you're on a diet. No problem! You can put together a delicious meal without a lot of fuss or time. Here, twelve hasty but tasty ways to get a good meal on the table.

1. Buy a ready-made rotisserie chicken. You can serve it as an entrée by itself or use the meat for fajitas, a casserole, a quick soup, a stir-fry, or a salad topping.

2. Grab bags of precut, prewashed veggies. You can find these either in the produce aisle or at the salad bar. Bring them home and toss them in a bowl for an easy salad.

3. Put shrimp on the menu. It takes only a few minutes to cook shrimp, and it's an incredibly tasty way to add variety to your meals. Pick some up at the fish counter or from the frozen food section.

4. Buy boil-in-a-bag rice. It can be prepared in just ten minutes, and today it comes in healthy whole-grain and brown varieties.

5. Get out your wok. Stir-fried dishes come together quickly, and they're loaded with healthy veggies and protein. No time to chop? Use those prewashed and cut bags of veggies.

6. Eat breakfast for dinner. Oatmeal, high-fiber cereal, and eggs are healthy, filling, and can be made in a few minutes flat.

7. Make takeout slimming. Order steamed veggies and plain brown rice from the Chinese restaurant or veggie sushi (brown rice if you can) and miso soup from the Japanese place. Restaurant fare won't derail your diet if you know what to choose.

8. Cook up frozen veggies like broccoli or spinach and cover with low-sugar jarred pasta sauce. Sprinkle on some Parmesan cheese and you're set.

9. Eat fast food. Yes, you read that right! Just don't eat it more than once a week, and make sure to order the smallest and least fatty items. For example, the Taco Bell bean burrito has 370 calories and twelve grams of fat, low by fast-food standards. Small burgers are also in this range. Before you hit the drive-through, visit the fast-food chain's website for calorie and other nutrition information. Better yet, keep a list in your wallet of the least diet-damaging options from each of the restaurants you visit often.

10. Look at your leftovers. It's easy to ignore those foil-covered dishes in your refrigerator, but you can actually whip up a quick, tasty meal with them. I love eating leftovers because it serves a dual purpose: It cleans out my refrigerator and feeds me well for little money.

11. Feel like a kid again and enjoy a simple peanut butter and jelly sandwich on whole-grain bread. You can also try natural peanut butter and honey or add some sliced bananas. Talk about comfort food!

12. Reach for the pasta. Most varieties boil up in twelve minutes or less and, if you opt for the whole wheat variety, are nutritious, too. Add a dash of olive oil or sprinkle of cheese and you've got a yummy meal in half the time it takes for a pizza delivery to arrive.

My Daily Dozen Sunday Checklist

	WEEK ONE	WEEK TWO	WEEK THREE
I ate my Daily Dozen Foods			
VEGGIE			
VEGGIE			
VEGGIE			
FRUIT			
FRUIT			
FRUIT			
PROTEIN			
PROTEIN			
PROTEIN			
HEALTHY GRAIN			
HEALTHY GRAIN			
HEALTHY FAT			
EIGHT 8-OUNCE GLASSES OF WATER			
I did my Daily Dozen exercises			
I did some of my weekly twelve miles of cardio (write how many miles)			
I did some fidget-cisers today (write how many)			

Twelve Ballet-Inspired Barre Exercises

While most of us weren't born with the lovely, long legs of a prima ballerina, we can definitely get our leg muscles looking leaner with these simple exercises. This is a 12-minute sequence of toning exercises that I have selected from my new DVD, *Body Makeover Mix*, that will tone your thighs and lift your seat. The following moves are great because you can do them anywhere—all you need is a chair to hold on to for balance. So what are you waiting for? Gorgeous dancer's legs are only a few pliés away!

1. Leg Swings

Get a beautiful dancer's body.

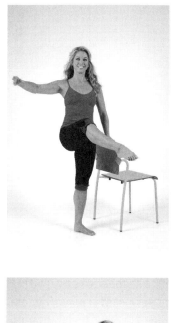

▸ Stand with your left side facing a chair and your left hand resting on it. Bring your legs together with your heels touching and toes pointing out on a diagonal. Extend your right arm out to the side at shoulder height. Lift the right leg up off the floor in front of you to hip height and turn it out to the side slightly while bending it.

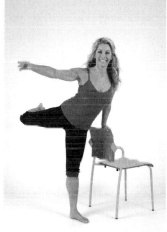

▸ Swing your right leg back behind you. Keep your back nice and straight, zip up those abs, and squeeze your buttocks as you swing the leg. Return to the start position and repeat. Time: 30 seconds on each leg.

2. Back Stretch

A wonderful way to elongate and stretch your spine, giving space to each vertebra.

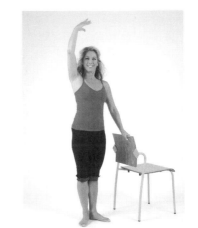

▸ Stand with your left side facing a chair and your left hand resting on it. Bring your legs together with your heels touching but your toes pointing out on a diagonal. Extend your right arm up toward the ceiling.

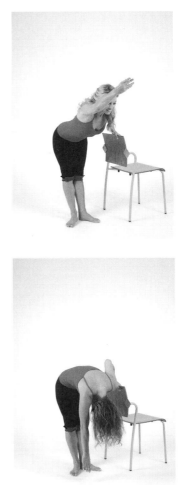

▸ Bend your upper body forward with a flat back. Reach your hand to the floor and let your head and neck release.

▸ Round your back, bring your navel to your spine, and now roll up one vertebra at a time. Go slowly and take your time rolling up to start position. You can probably do about three of these correctly in a minute. Time: 1 minute.

3. Plié
Firm those inner thighs fast!

▸ Stand with your left side facing a chair and your left hand resting on it, with toes turned out slightly and heels together and lifted a few inches off the floor. Bring your right arm out to the side at shoulder height. Bend your knees into a low plié as you press your heels together like glue. Squeeze your inner thighs as you return to standing. Keep your back straight and zip up those abs the entire time. Time: 1 minute.

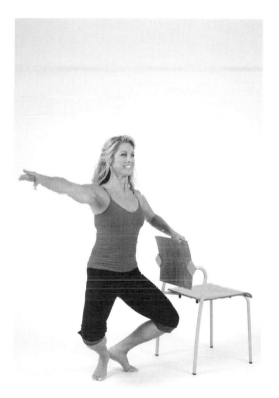

4. Tuck

Reshaping your lower half has never been easier! This is a small, focused move that works.

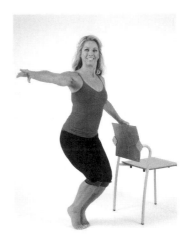

▸ Holding on to the chair with your left arm, turn your body on a diagonal toward the chair. Bring your legs and feet together, lift your heels several inches off the ground, and bend your knees. Extend your right arm out to the side at shoulder height.

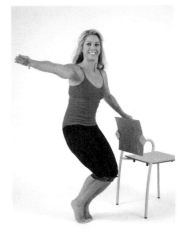

▸ With your inner thighs squeezing together, alternate tucking your pelvis forward and back. The higher the heels come off the floor, the trimmer the thighs. Time: 1 minute.

▸ CHALLENGE: Stand in the same position but hold on to the back of the chair with both hands. Lean back slightly as you tuck your pelvis.

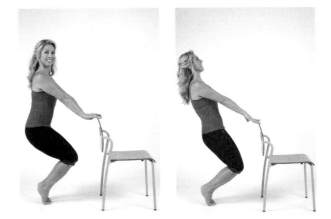

5. Hamstring

Tighten and tone the backs of the thighs and lift your seat.

▸ Turn the chair so that you are facing the seat. Stand with your feet and legs together and lean forward from the waist. Place your palms on the seat of the chair and lift your right leg straight behind you so it's one line from your right leg to your head.

▸ Flexing your foot, bend and straighten your right leg, pulling your heel to your rear. Keep your back strong and navel pulled toward your spine the whole time. Time: 30 seconds per leg. Round your back to stretch it out. Then switch legs and repeat.

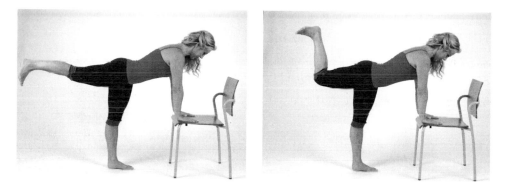

6. Curl-Ups

Shape your way to thinner thighs and a toned flat tummy.

▸ Kneel on the floor and sit on your heels.

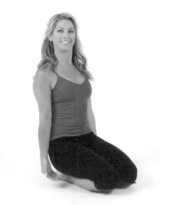

▸ Keep your back nice and straight. Tilt your pelvis up and lift your buttocks off your rear as you scoop your abs up and in.

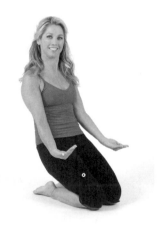

▸ Sit all the way up and extend your arms out at shoulder height. Then push down with your arms as you sit back on your heels. Time: 1 minute.

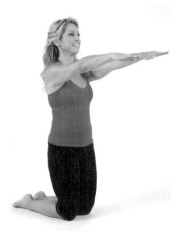

7. The Pretzel

Lift those buns and transform your bottom half.

▶ Sit with your right leg bent in front of you and your left leg bent behind you. Place your hands on the floor in front of you.

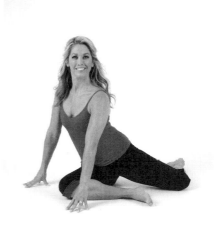

▶ Lift the left leg off the floor just an inch or two behind you. Now pulse by lifting and lowering the bent leg. This pulse is a very small movement that focuses on the deeper muscles. Time: 30 seconds. Switch legs and repeat.

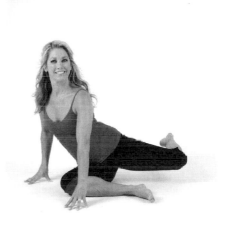

8. Starfish

I love this one because it targets the legs and contours the waistline.

▸ Sit with your left leg bent in front of you on the floor and your right leg bent upward to the side over your left leg, with the toe pointed on the floor. Place the palm of your left hand on the floor and bend your right arm, placing the elbow on your right knee.

▸ Lift your hips up and extend your right leg straight out at hip height and your right arm straight alongside your head in one line, so you're balancing on your left knee and hand. Time: 30 seconds. Switch sides and repeat.

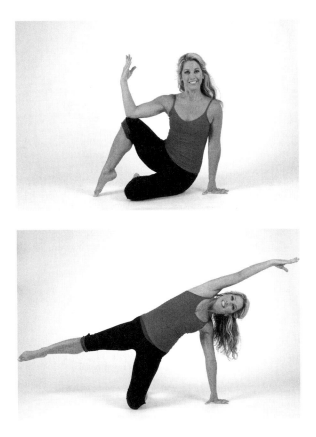

9. Bridge
Reshape your rear and flatten your abs all at once!

▸ Lie on your back with your knees bent and feet flat on the floor about hip-width apart. Extend your arms straight alongside your body. Lift your heels and hips up off the ground.

▸ Tuck your pelvis up and down. Time: 1 minute.

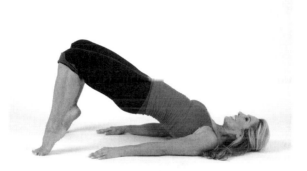

▸ CHALLENGE: Bring your legs together while tucking, which targets your inner thighs, too.

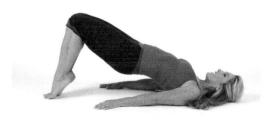

10. Leg Scissors
Create a bikini-worthy belly!

▶ Lie on your back with your legs extended straight up toward the ceiling. Place your arms by your sides with your palms on the floor and lift your head, neck, and shoulders off the floor. Slowly lower your right leg down so it hovers about four to five inches off the floor. Then as you bring it back up toward the ceiling, lower your left leg. Flatten out your tummy and point your toes. Time: 1 minute.

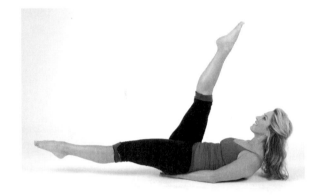

▶ CHALLENGE: Place your hands behind your head.

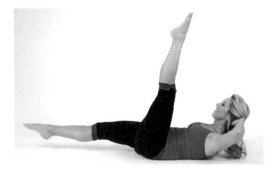

11. Cross Lift

Melt those "love" handles that we hate.

▶ Begin in the same position you are in for the leg scissors, with your hands behind your head. As you bring the left leg up toward the ceiling, extend your right arm up toward it. Then as you bring your right leg up toward the ceiling, extend your left arm up toward it. Time: 1 minute.

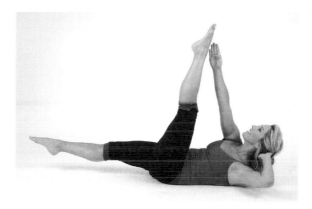

▶ CHALLENGE: Twist your upper body and opposite shoulder to the opposite leg.

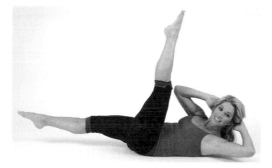

12. Can Can

Oh yes, you can can get great abs!

▸ Sit on the floor with your hands behind your back and your legs bent and lifted off the floor. Straighten the legs as you bring them to the left. Then bend them and straighten them as you bring them to the right. Keep alternating. Time: 1 minute.

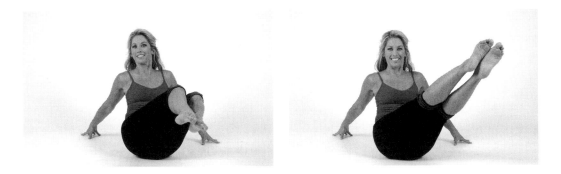

▸ CHALLENGE: Sit in a V-position with your legs straight and your arms extended straight toward your legs.

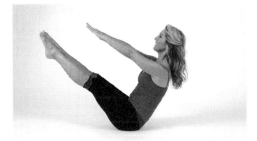

TWELVE MEALS YOU CAN MAKE IN ABOUT TWELVE MINUTES

BREAKFASTS

Western Scramble

This scramble has a kitchen sink's worth of ingredients—meat, cheese, and veggies galore. If your family doesn't like bell peppers, you can get creative with substitutions: Spinach or zucchini would also be good. If they don't like ham, add crumbled-up cooked turkey sausage instead. And try adding some herbs—some flat-leaf parsley would be tasty, as would basil or thyme (or sage, if you're using sausage). If you can cook the potatoes the night before, the dish will come together even more quickly.

1 small red or Idaho potato, cut into ½-inch cubes
1 tablespoon canola oil
1 medium yellow onion, coarsely chopped
1 medium red bell pepper, coarsely chopped (or substitute spinach or zucchini)
½ medium green bell pepper, coarsely chopped
½ cup extra-lean ham, finely chopped (or substitute crumbled-up cooked turkey sausage)
2 large eggs plus 4 large egg whites
2 tablespoons low-fat cottage cheese
½ teaspoon freshly ground black pepper
Pinch of salt

(continued on next page)

Put the potato in a medium saucepan. Add cold water to barely cover. Bring to a boil over high heat. Reduce the heat to medium, partially cover, and cook until tender, about 7 minutes. Drain.

Heat the oil in a large nonstick skillet over medium-high heat. Add the onion and bell peppers and cook, stirring often, until the peppers are tender and the onion is lightly golden, about 8 minutes. Stir in the ham and potato and cook, stirring often, until the mixture is just starting to brown, about 2 minutes.

In a medium bowl, beat the eggs, egg whites, cottage cheese, black pepper, and salt until well blended. Pour the egg mixture into the skillet over the vegetables and ham. Reduce the heat to medium and cook, turning often with a heat-proof spatula, until the eggs are just set, about 2 minutes.

Serves 4

NUTRITIONAL INFORMATION (PER SERVING)
Calories: 150 kcal
Total Fat: 8 g
Saturated Fat: 1 g
Total Carbohydrate: 14 g
Protein: 13 g
Sodium: 341 mg
Fiber: 2 g

Breakfast Burritos

One of the best things about these breakfast burritos is that they can be made to order! People who like spicy food can ramp up the flavor with some hot sauce, people who aren't dieting can add a little low-fat cheese, and people who are following my plan can have a breakfast with plenty of zip but not a lot of calories!

For the salsa:
½ cup firm red and/or yellow cherry tomatoes, quartered
½ ripe avocado, finely chopped
1 tablespoon fresh lime juice
¼ teaspoon ground cumin
Pinch of salt

For the burritos:
4 whole wheat tortillas (7½-inch diameter)
½ cup fat-free refried beans
4 large eggs
2 tablespoons water
⅛ teaspoon salt
⅛ teaspoon freshly ground black pepper

To make the salsa: In a small bowl, gently mix the tomatoes, avocado, lime juice, cumin, and pinch of salt. Cover and set aside.

To make the burritos: Warm the tortillas in the microwave or a conventional oven according to the package directions. Cover with foil to keep warm. Place the beans in a small microwave-safe bowl, cover, and microwave on high for 45 seconds, or until hot. Keep warm.

In a medium bowl, whisk the eggs, water, salt, and pepper until well blended. Coat a medium nonstick skillet with cooking spray. Heat over medium heat. Add the eggs and scramble until cooked but still moist.

One at a time, spread each warm tortilla with about 2 tablespoons of the beans and a quarter of the eggs. Top each with about 2 tablespoons of salsa, reserving the rest to serve at the table. Roll up the tortillas, folding in the sides. Serve right away, with the remaining salsa.

Serves 4

NUTRITIONAL INFORMATION (PER SERVING)
Calories: 290 kcal
Total Fat: 12 g
Saturated Fat: 3 g
Total Carbohydrate: 32 g
Protein: 13 g
Sodium: 480 mg
Fiber: 6 g

LUNCHES

Shrimp with Vegetables & Old Bay Vinaigrette

This is such a light and refreshing dish, and it's so healthy, too! This is from my friend Laurie Potts, the top chef of the world famous Wildhorse Saloon in Nashville, Tennessee. Enjoy this meal with your girlfriends—they will love it!

For the shrimp:
2 cups yellow tomatoes
2 cups red tomatoes
1 cup julienned red onion
2 cups cucumbers
1 pound boiled shrimp

For the vinaigrette:
1 cup red wine vinegar
2 cups olive oil
½ cup Old Bay Seasoning
2 tablespoons chopped fresh dill
Salt and pepper, to taste

Combine the shrimp and vegetables in a bowl and mix. Set aside. Mix the dressing ingredients in a small bowl. Pour over the shrimp and veggies. Refrigerate any remaining dressing.

Serves 4

NUTRITIONAL INFORMATION (PER SERVING)
Calories: 290 kcal
Total Fat: 16 g
Saturated Fat: 2.5 g
Total Carbohydrate: 11 g
Protein: 26 g
Sodium: 280 mg
Fiber: 3 g

Chutney Chicken Wrap

I love this quick and easy chicken wrap, and the taste of chutney makes it so scrumptious and exotic. If you happen to be making a roasted chicken dinner, consider making a second chicken and saving some of the meat for this terrific wrap. Or use some rotisserie chicken from the market.

2 tablespoons chutney
¼ cup low-fat mayonnaise
4 low-fat tortillas (8-inch diameter)
4 large red-lettuce leaves
2 cups shredded cooked chicken breast or 8 ounces sliced smoked turkey breast
1 cup finely shredded carrots

Mix the chutney and mayonnaise in a small bowl. If you have time, cover and re-frigerate for 20 minutes for the flavors to develop.

Spread a scant 1½ tablespoons of the chutney mixture on each tortilla. Top each with a lettuce leaf, ½ cup chicken or 2 ounces turkey, and ¼ cup carrots. Roll the wraps tightly and cut in half diagonally.

Serves 4

NUTRITIONAL INFORMATION (PER WRAP)
Calories: 269 kcal
Total Fat: 6 g
Saturated Fat: 2 g
Total Carbohydrate: 30 g
Protein: 23 g
Sodium: 471 mg
Fiber: 2 g

Black Bean Soup

This is one of my husband's favorite soups. Plus, black beans are so good for you. I make this for my family quite often because it lasts in the refrigerator for days. Just heat it up and serve this sure-to-please soup that is easy to prepare.

1 teaspoon olive oil
1 medium carrot, chopped
1 clove garlic, finely chopped
¼ cup diced onion
¼ cup diced red bell pepper
1 teaspoon cumin
Pinch of red pepper flakes
Pinch of salt
1 cup water
½ can (15 ounces) black beans, rinsed and drained
½ cup reduced-sodium chicken broth
¼ cup chopped fresh cilantro
1 teaspoon freshly squeezed lime juice

Heat the oil in saucepan or soup pot; add the carrot, garlic, onion, and bell pepper and sauté for 10 to 12 minutes until softened. Add the cumin, red pepper flakes, and salt, followed by the water, black beans, and chicken broth. Bring the mixture to a boil, reduce the heat to low, and simmer for 12 minutes. Ladle the soup into a blender and puree until smooth. Return the soup to the pot to reheat, stir in the cilantro and lime juice—and serve.

Serves 1

NUTRITIONAL INFORMATION (PER SERVING)
Calories: 250 kcal
Total Fat: 6 g
Saturated Fat: 1 g
Total Carbohydrate: 41 g
Protein: 11 g
Sodium: 814 mg
Fiber: 14 g

Country Garden Gazpacho with Garlic Croutons

It's a good idea to make this gazpacho first thing in the morning or the night before so it can chill in the fridge while the flavors develop and the spicy fresh flavors meld. You can serve it for lunch or with some salad or steamed veggies for a light, no-meat dinner.

2 large cloves garlic
3 large ripe tomatoes, peeled and cut into chunks
1 medium cucumber, peeled and cut into chunks
½ large red bell pepper, cut into chunks
½ cup chopped red or white sweet onion
1 cup tomato juice
1 tablespoon fresh lemon juice
¼ teaspoon salt
⅛ teaspoon ground red pepper
1 tablespoon extra-virgin olive oil
2 slices whole wheat bread, cut into ½-inch cubes

Drop 1 garlic clove through the feed tube of a running food processor and process until finely chopped. In batches, add the tomatoes, cucumber, bell pepper, and onion; process until pureed. Pour into a large bowl. Stir in the tomato juice, lemon juice, salt, and red pepper. Cover and refrigerate for about 2 hours, until well chilled.

Meanwhile, smash the remaining garlic clove with the flat side of a chef's knife or a meat mallet. Place the garlic and oil in a medium nonstick skillet over medium-low heat. Cook, turning and pressing down on the garlic, until golden, about 4 minutes. Discard the garlic.

Add the bread cubes to the garlic oil and cook, stirring, until browned and crisp, 2 to 3 minutes. Transfer the croutons to a bowl and let cool. To serve, stir the soup and ladle it into bowls. Top each serving with some of the croutons. You're going to love it!

Serves 2

(continued on next page)

NUTRITIONAL INFORMATION (PER 1¼-CUP SERVING)

Calories: 130 kcal

Total Fat: 4.5 g

Saturated Fat: 1 g

Total Carbohydrate: 21 g

Protein: 4 g

Sodium: 450 mg

Fiber: 4 g

Wild Rice & Asparagus Salad

This is a great make-ahead salad. I prepare the rice in advance and chill it until I have time to chop up the veggies. It's also a great side dish at dinner.

4 cups wild rice (or any rice)
2 bunches asparagus
1 red bell pepper, diced
1 green bell pepper, diced
1 cup diced red onion
8 ounces arugula
1 cup chopped fresh basil
Store-bought low-fat Italian or balsamic dressing

Cook the rice according to package directions, then cool. Drop the asparagus in boiling water for 2 minutes and then drunk it in ice water to cool. Discard the bottom 2 inches of each stalk (because it is tough), and cut the remaining asparagus into 1-inch pieces on the bias. Mix all ingredients together and add your favorite low-fat Italian or balsamic dressing!

Serves 4

NUTRITIONAL INFORMATION (PER SERVING)
Calories: 239 kcal
Total Fat: 2 g
Saturated Fat: 0 g
Total Carbohydrate: 48 g
Protein: 15 g
Sodium: 27 mg
Fiber: 7 g

Broccoli & Cauliflower Salad

This crunchy salad is as healthy as it gets! If you want to eat "raw," this would be a great lunch. You get veggies, berries, and protein with the sunflower seeds. And it's so easy to prepare.

1 bunch broccoli, cut into bite-size pieces
1 head cauliflower, cut into bite-size pieces
½ red onion, julienned
¼ cup dried berries (I use cranberries)
¼ cup sunflower seeds
2 tablespoons store-bought low-fat coleslaw dressing

Mix all the ingredients together in a bowl. Add coleslaw dressing and enjoy! Wasn't that easy?

Serves 4

NUTRITIONAL INFORMATION (PER SERVING)
Calories: 190 kcal
Total Fat: 7 g
Saturated Fat: 1 g
Total Carbohydrate: 27 g
Protein: 9 g
Sodium: 493 mg
Fiber: 8 g

DINNERS

Shrimp Shack Special

You can buy the shrimp already peeled and deveined, or you can buy them fresh at the fishmonger and set one of your kids up to do the dirty work. If you're using frozen shrimp, which is perfectly okay, thaw them in a bowl of cool water, drain them, and pat them dry. Using premade low-fat coleslaw mix is another time saver. And if you're really feeling pressed for time, you can use bottled cocktail sauce instead of making it fresh.

For the shrimp:
1 pound peeled and deveined medium shrimp, thawed if frozen
2 tablespoons fresh lemon juice
1 teaspoon hot pepper sauce
1 teaspoon extra-virgin olive oil
⅛ teaspoon salt (optional)

For the slaw:
2 tablespoons reduced-fat mayonnaise
2 tablespoons reduced-fat sour cream
1 tablespoon cider vinegar
1 teaspoon chili powder
¼–½ teaspoon hot pepper sauce, to taste
⅛ teaspoon salt
3 cups prepared coleslaw mix
1 can (15 ounces) pinto beans, drained and rinsed

For the shrimp sauce: (You can buy this if you're time-pressed)
¼ cup ketchup
1–2 tablespoons prepared white horseradish
1 tablespoon fresh lemon juice

To make the shrimp: Coat a rimmed baking sheet with cooking spray. Place the shrimp in a mound on the pan and mix with the lemon juice, pepper sauce, oil, and salt (if using). Spread out on the pan. Let stand for 10 minutes while you prepare the slaw and the sauce.

To make the slaw: In a salad bowl, mix the mayonnaise, sour cream, vinegar, chili powder, pepper sauce, and salt. Add the coleslaw mix and beans and toss to mix well.

To make the sauce: In a small bowl, mix the ketchup, horseradish, and lemon juice.

Preheat the broiler. Broil the shrimp 3 to 4 inches from the heat until pink and just opaque in the thickest part, about 5 minutes.

Serve the shrimp with the sauce and the slaw.

Serves 4

NUTRITIONAL INFORMATION (PER SERVING)
Calories: 240 kcal
Total Fat: 6 g
Saturated Fat: 1.5 g
Total Carbohydrate: 23 g
Protein: 25 g
Sodium: 660 mg
Fiber: 5 g

Slim Sloppy Joes

I can't tell you how often I've heard this: "I can't make diet food for my family, because they won't eat it." Thing is, nothing on my plan is "diet" food per se; it's regular food that I've trimmed calories from by using lower-fat ingredients and bulked up with extra veggies. It tastes the same, so if you don't spill the secret, no one at your table will ever know you're looking out for their health!

¾ pound lean ground beef (round or sirloin) or ground turkey
1 teaspoon canola oil
1 large green bell pepper, chopped
2 cans (8 ounces each) tomato sauce
⅔ cup frozen corn kernels
2 tablespoons ketchup
1 tablespoon cider vinegar

(continued on next page)

1 teaspoon sugar
¼ teaspoon freshly ground black pepper
Whole wheat hamburger buns

Coat a large nonstick skillet with cooking spray and heat over medium-high heat. Crumble in the beef and cook, stirring often, until it loses its pink color, about 5 minutes. Drain the beef in a colander and wipe out the skillet.

In the same skillet, heat the oil over medium heat. Add the bell pepper and cook, stirring often, until tender, about 3 minutes. Return the beef to the skillet and stir in the tomato sauce, corn, ketchup, vinegar, sugar, and black pepper. Bring just to a boil. Reduce the heat and simmer until slightly thickened, about 10 minutes.

Serve on whole wheat hamburger buns with add-ons like chopped onion, pickled peppers, pickle slices, grated low-fat cheese, tomato slices, or whatever other toppings you like. *Note:* This recipe makes enough for two meals, so put half in the freezer for a busy day.

Makes 4 cups

NUTRITIONAL INFORMATION (PER ½-CUP SERVING)
Calories: 150 kcal
Total Fat: 5 g
Saturated Fat: 1 g
Total Carbohydrate: 21 g
Protein: 12 g
Sodium: 470 mg
Fiber: 3 g

Lime-Grilled Chicken with Cuban Salsa

I love this recipe because it's festive enough to serve to company, and just as perfect when you make it for your family as a special treat. It's light and a little spicy—ideal for the summer, when you can throw the chicken on the grill, or the fall, when a broiler is the way to go. If you like, turn up the heat with more jalapeño! If you want to tone it down, use less (make sure you remove the seeds, too, which are extra-spicy!). Allow a little extra time to let the chicken marinate before cooking—twelve minutes will do it. You can also marinate the chicken in a resealable plastic bag overnight in the fridge (just bring it back to room temperature before using) and make the salsa the night before. Then all you'll have to do to finish dinner is cook the chicken and some brown rice, and put together a spinach salad.

For the salsa:
1/2 can (15 ounces) black beans
1 ripe mango, finely diced
3 tablespoons chopped red onion
3 tablespoons lime juice
2 tablespoons chopped fresh cilantro
1/2 jalapeño pepper, finely diced (optional)

For the chicken:
4 boneless, skinless chicken breast halves
2 teaspoons grated lime peel
2 tablespoons fresh lime juice
2 teaspoons canola oil
1/2 teaspoon salt
1/4 teaspoon freshly ground black pepper

To make the salsa: In a medium bowl, stir together the beans, mango, onion, lime juice, cilantro, and jalapeño.

To make the chicken: Preheat your grill or broiler. If you're using a broiler, coat the broiler pan with cooking spray. Place the chicken in a shallow dish. Add the lime peel, lime juice, oil, salt, and pepper, and rub the mixture into the chicken. Cover and let stand for 15 minutes.

Place the chicken on the grill rack or broiler pan and cook 4 inches from the heat, turning once, until the chicken is no longer pink in the thickest part, 10 to 12 minutes. Serve the chicken with the salsa; if desired, slice the chicken into strips before serving.

Serves 4

(*continued on next page*)

NUTRITIONAL INFORMATION (PER SERVING)
Calories: 290 kcal
Total Fat: 5 g
Saturated Fat: 1 g
Total Carbohydrate: 22 g
Protein: 37 g
Sodium: 620 mg
Fiber: 5 g

Artichoke with Lemon Thyme Vinaigrette

I love artichokes and so do my daughters. They are fun to eat, too. We like to dip them in this Lemon Thyme Vinaigrette. Whenever I make this vinaigrette, I make a lot so I can keep it in the fridge for salads, too!

4 fresh artichokes with bottom leaves trimmed and stems peeled
Lemon juice
Salt
Olive oil
Pepper

For the Lemon Thyme Vinaigrette:
1 cup fresh squeezed lemon juice
2 cups olive oil
3 tablespoons chopped garlic
3 tablespoons shallots
3 tablespoons fresh thyme
Salt and pepper, to taste

Cut the artichokes in half and remove the inner thistle with a vegetable peeler. Place the artichokes in lemon water until you are ready to cook them. Boil them in salted lemon water for 9 minutes (or longer if you like them really soft), then remove from the water and brush with olive oil, salt, and pepper before grilling for 3 minutes on each side.

To make the Lemon Thyme Vinaigrette: Whisk together the lemon juice, olive oil, garlic, shallots, fresh thyme, salt, and pepper. Serve half of the dressing with the artichokes. Refrigerate remaining dressing for other uses.

Serves 4

NUTRITIONAL INFORMATION (PER SERVING)
Calories: 241 kcal
Total Fat: 2 g
Saturated Fat: 0 g
Total Carbohydrate: 59 g
Protein: 10 g
Sodium: 310 mg
Fiber: 14 g

SHOPPING LISTS

I've put together shopping lists for each week, but be sure to check your kitchen and cross off the things you already have before you head to the store. I like to go to local farmer's markets, where you can pick what you like and only buy as much as you need. It's also usually cheaper and fresher. You also may find you have some ingredients left over from a previous week, but I've listed everything just so you know what you'll need.

Week One Shopping List

DAIRY/EGGS
Butter spray, 1 bottle
Cheese, nonfat cottage, women:
    4 ounces; men: 16 ounces
Cheese, feta, crumbled, 1 package
Cheese, goat, 2.5 ounces, 1 package
Cheese, low-fat Monterey Jack,
    shredded, 1 package
Cheese, Parmesan, grated,
    1 package
Eggs, 1 dozen
Milk, skim, ½ gallon
Sour cream, light, 6 ounces
Yogurt, nonfat vanilla, 8 ounces

MEAT/FISH
Chicken breast, boneless and skinless,
    women: 8 ounces; men: 1 pound
Fish, salmon, women: 3 ounces; men:
    5 ounces
Shrimp, 8 jumbo
Steak, flank, 4 ounces
Turkey breast, roasted, 8 ounces

BAKERY
Bread, sprouted grain, 1 loaf
Bread, whole wheat, 1 loaf
Pita, whole wheat, 1 package
Tortilla, whole grain, 1 package

PRODUCE

Apples, women: 5; men: 6

Apples, Granny Smith, women: 1; men: 2

Avocado, 1

Banana, 1

Blueberries, women: 2 pints; men: 3 pints

Grapefruit, women: 2; men: 3

Kiwi, 1

Lemon, 1

Limes, 2

Mango, 1

Melon, cantaloupe, 1

Oranges, 5

Pears, women: 2; men: 3

Pineapple, 1

Pomegranate, 1

Raspberries, 2 pints

Strawberries, women: 1 pint; men: 1 quart

Asparagus, 1 bunch

Bell pepper, red, 2

Bell pepper, yellow, 2

Broccoli slaw, pre-shredded, 1 package

Carrots, 2 pounds

Celery, 1 bunch

Corn, 1 small ear

Cucumber, 1

Greens/lettuce, mixed, 1 package

Mushrooms, button, 8-ounce package

Onion, red, 1

Peas, snow, 8-ounce package

Potato, Idaho, 1

Potato, sweet, 1

Shallot, 1 large

Spinach, baby, 1 package

Tomato, beefsteak, 1

Tomatoes, plum, 5–6

Basil, fresh, 1 package

Cilantro, fresh, 1 bunch

Garlic, 1 bulb

Rosemary, fresh, 1 package

FROZEN

Vegetables, frozen mixed, 1 package (1 cup)

Waffles, whole grain, frozen, 1 package

MISCELLANEOUS GROCERY (SNACKS, DRY GOODS, CANNED)

Cereal, bran flakes, 1 box

Oatmeal, 1 container

Cranberries, dried, 8-ounce package

Nuts, almonds, raw, 1 pound

Seeds, flaxseed, 1 pound

Fruit spread, all natural, 1 jar

Peanut butter, natural, 1 jar

Syrup, maple, 1 bottle

Crackers, rice or Sesmark, 1 box

Rice, brown, 1 pound

Spaghetti, whole wheat, 1 pound

Soup, Amy's Organic Black Bean
   Vegetable Soup, 1 can
Soup, low-sodium chicken broth, 1 can
Tuna, canned in water, 1 can
   (6 ounces)

Dressing, champagne vinaigrette,
   1 bottle
Honey, 1 bottle

Mayonnaise, light, 1 jar
Mustard, Dijon, 1 jar
Mustard, honey, 1 jar
Oil, canola, 1 bottle
Oil, olive, 1 bottle
Salsa, 1 jar
Soy sauce, reduced sodium, 1 bottle
Vinegar, balsamic, 1 bottle

Seasoning, grill, 1 container

Week Two Shopping List

DAIRY/EGGS
Cheese, Cabot reduced-fat cheddar,
   1 package
Cheese, nonfat cottage, 32 ounces
Cheese, low-fat feta, crumbled,
   1 package
Cheese, part-skim mozzarella string,
   1 package
Eggs, 1 dozen
Juice, orange, 1 pint
Milk, skim, 1 gallon
Yogurt, Greek, nonfat, 16 ounces
Yogurt, nonfat, 32 ounces

MEAT/FISH
Chicken breast, boneless, skinless,
   women: 4 ounces; men: 8 ounces
Chicken breast, ground, 4 ounces
Chicken breast, roasted, 3 ounces
Fish, halibut, 4 ounces
Fish, mahi mahi, 4 ounces

Fish, red snapper, 3 ounces
Pork tenderloin, roasted, 4 ounces
Turkey breast, roasted, 5 ounces

BAKERY
Bread, whole wheat, 1 loaf
English muffins, whole grain,
   1 package
Tortillas, corn, 1 package
Tortillas, sprouted grain, 1 package
Tortillas, whole wheat, 1 package

PRODUCE
Apples, 4
Avocado, 1
Bananas, women: 1; men: 2
Blackberries, women: 2 pints; men:
   3 pints
Blueberries, women: 2 pints; men:
   3 pints
Grapes, green, 1 bunch

Grapes, red, 1 bunch
Kiwi, 1 (men only)
Mango, 1
Melon, 1
Orange, 1
Pear, 1
Pineapple, 1
Raspberries, women: 2 pints; men:
   3 pints
Strawberries, 1-pound container
Tangerine, 1

Asparagus, 2 bunches
Bell pepper, red, 1
Broccoli, 1 bunch
Cabbage, green, 1 medium-size
   head
Carrots, baby, 1 bag
Cauliflower, 1 head
Celery, 1 bunch
Cucumber, 2
Cucumber, English, 1
Eggplant, 1 medium-size
Greens/lettuce, mixed, 1-pound
   package
Lettuce, arugula, 8 ounces
Lettuce, iceberg, 1 small head
Onion, red, 1
Peas, snow, women: ½ pound;
   men: 1 pound
Scallion, 1 bunch
Shallot, 1 large
Spinach, baby, 8-ounce package
Tomatoes, 3
Tomatoes, cherry, 1 pint

Garlic, 1 bulb

FROZEN
Berries, frozen mixed, 1 pound
Vegetables, frozen mixed, 1 bag
Waffles, whole grain, frozen,
   1 package

MISCELLANEOUS GROCERY
(SNACKS, DRY GOODS, CANNED)
Hummus, 1 container

Barley, quick-cooking, 1 box
Oatmeal, 1 container
Oatmeal, Irish (steel-cut oats),
   1 box

Bread crumbs, panko, 1 container

Nuts, almonds, 1 pound (men only)
Nuts, walnuts, 1 pound
Raisins, 1 large box
Seeds, ground flaxseed, 1 pound
Seeds, sesame seeds, black, 1 container

Granola bars, 1 box

Peanut butter, natural, 1 jar

Couscous, whole wheat, 1 box
Crackers, whole wheat, 1 package
Lentils, green or brown, dry, 1 bag
Pretzels, 1 bag
Quinoa, 1 pound
Rice, brown, 1 pound

Beans, black, canned, 1 can
Chickpeas, canned, 1 can
Corn, canned, 1 can
Red peppers, roasted, 1 large jar

Soup, low-sodium chicken broth,
    1 can
Soup, low-sodium lentil, 1 can

Salsa, 1 jar

Chili sauce, hot, 1 jar
Dressing, light honey mustard, 1 jar

Dressing, vinaigrette, 1 bottle
Honey, 1 container
Lemon juice, 1 container
Oil, canola, 16-ounce bottle
Oil, olive, 16-ounce bottle
Oil, sesame, 8-ounce bottle
Teriyaki sauce, 1 bottle
Vinegar, balsamic, one 32-ounce bottle
Vinegar, red wine, 1 bottle

Cinnamon, 1 container
Cinnamon sticks, 1 container
Seasoning, lemon pepper, 1 container

Week Three Shopping List

DAIRY/EGGS
Cheese, fresh mozzarella, 1 package
Cheese, grated Parmesan
Cheese, light Jarlsberg
Cheese, low-fat feta, crumbled,
    1 package
Cheese, low-fat shredded, 1 package
Cheese, part-skim mozzarella string,
    1 small package
Cheese, part-skim ricotta, one 8-ounce
    container
Eggs, 1 dozen
Juice, orange, 1 pint
Milk, skim, 1 quart
Yogurt, Greek, 1 small container
Yogurt, nonfat vanilla, 1 large
    container (32 ounces)

MEAT
Chicken breast, boneless and skinless,
    1 pound
Fish, salmon, 5 ounces
Ham, lean (or lean turkey breast or
    Canadian bacon), 1 ounce
Steak, flank, 4 ounces
Turkey breast, ground, 3 ounces

BAKERY
Bread, whole wheat, 1 loaf
English muffins, whole grain,
    1 package
Pita, whole wheat, 1 package

PRODUCE
Apples, 3
Bananas, 3
Grapefruit, 1

Grapes, red, 1 bunch
Kiwi, 1
Lemons, 2
Mango, 1
Melon, 1
Oranges, 3
Pears, 2
Pineapple, 1
Strawberries, 1-pound container
Tangerines, 2 (men only)

Bell pepper, red, 2
Bell pepper, yellow, 2
Broccoli, 2 bunches
Broccoli slaw, pre-shredded, 1 package
Cabbage, green, 1 medium-size head
Carrots, baby, 1 bag
Celery, 1 bunch
Cucumber, 1 large
Greens/lettuce, mixed, 1-pound
    package
Onions, red, 3
Potatoes, Idaho russet, 2
Scallions, 1 bunch
Spinach, baby, 1-pound package
Swiss chard, 1 large bunch
Tomato, 1
Tomatoes, cherry, 1 pint
Zucchini, 1 large

Basil, fresh, 1 bunch
Garlic, 1 bulb
Gingerroot, 1 small piece
Parsley, fresh, 1 bunch
Thyme, fresh, 1 package

FROZEN
Blueberries, frozen, 1 bag
Orange juice, frozen concentrate,
    1 can
Vegetables, frozen mixed, 1 bag

**MISCELLANEOUS GROCERY
(SNACKS, DRY GOODS, CANNED)**
Hummus, 1 container

Barley, quick-cooking, 1 box
Oatmeal, 1 box
Oatmeal, Irish (steel-cut oats),
    1 box

Chow mein noodles, crispy,
    1 container

Nuts, almonds, 1-pound bag
Nuts, walnuts, 1-pound bag
Raisins, 1 large box

Granola bars, 1 box

Peanut butter, natural, 16-ounce jar

Cereal, whole grain, 1 box
Cornmeal, 1 box
Crackers, whole wheat, 1 box
Pasta, whole wheat, 16-ounce bag
    (or box)
Quinoa, 1 box
Rice, brown, 1-pound bag

Pizza dough, whole wheat, 1 large

Salmon, canned in water, 1 can
Tuna, canned in water, 1 can,
    men only

Beans, black, canned, 1 can
Olives, black, canned, 1 can
Tomato paste, 1 small can
Tomato sauce, 16-ounce jar

Soup, low-sodium chicken broth,
    1 can
Soup, low-sodium minestrone, 1 can

Salsa, 1 jar
Jalapeño pepper, pickled, 1 jar

Capers, 1 small jar
Dressing, balsamic vinaigrette, 1 small
    bottle

Dressing, light ranch, 1 small bottle
Dressing, low-fat Italian, 1 bottle
Honey, 1 jar
Oil, canola, 16-ounce bottle
Oil, olive, 16-ounce bottle
Soy sauce, reduced sodium, 1 bottle
Vinegar, red wine, 1 small bottle

Basil, dried, 1 container
Bay leaves, 1 container
Chinese five-spice powder,
    1 container
Cinnamon, 1 container
Curry powder, 1 container
Oregano, dried, 1 container
    (or 1 bunch if fresh)
Red pepper flakes, 1 container

Sugar, brown, 1 box

RECIPE INDEX